Praise for *Somatic Internal Family Systems Therapy*

"With *Somatic Internal Family Systems Therapy*, Susan McConnell brilliantly weaves together science, clinical stories, and experiential practices to bring Somatic IFS to life for her reader. The deep wisdom she embodies from years of studying the bodymind is felt in each of the five practices that are the foundation of Somatic IFS and in her clear yet lyrical explanation of the body systems that inform each practice. Susan McConnell is an expert guide to learning to listen to somatic stories and finding the way to Embodied Self."

—DEB DANA, LCSW, author of *The Polyvagal Theory in Therapy: Engaging the Rhythm of Regulation*

"This excellent book takes a very interesting look at family systems therapy—from a very somatic perspective. The theory and method of Somatic IFS really comes alive through case vignettes, clinical examples, practical exercises, and reflections. Referencing many other body-oriented practices, therapists, and researchers, this book offers an up-to-date, pragmatic method of working somatically with people: a methodology which other psychotherapists—especially those from non-somatic disciplines—can readily learn from."

—COURTENAY YOUNG, UK body psychotherapist, editor of the *International Journal of Psychotherapy*

"Susan McConnell writes from her heart and her embodied experience, as a counselor and an explorer in the somatic world. This book is an expression of her whole life and career, and yet the ideas are kept alive and honest through the immediacy of her practices—in psychotherapy, in somatics, and in spirituality. I hope that this book is read widely both in and beyond the IFS community."

—SUSAN APOSHYAN, LPC, author of *Body-Mind Psychotherapy: Principles, Techniques, and Practical Applications*

"A brilliant psychotherapeutic integration of mind and body by a wise and experienced somatic practitioner who weaves Internal Family Systems therapy into a method that facilitates the achievement of an Embodied Self. Through descriptions and explanations of the five practices of Somatic IFS, illustrative case examples, and guided practices, the author connects the gifts of ancient medicine and contemporary neuroscience to the benefit of professionals and laypersons alike. A unique and timely book."

—MARCEL A. DUCLOS, LCMHC, LPC, ACS, Diplomate, AMHCA, certified Core Energetics therapist, certified IFS therapist

Somatic
Internal Family Systems
Therapy

Somatic
Internal Family Systems
Therapy

Awareness, Breath, Resonance, Movement, and Touch in Practice

Susan McConnell

Foreword by Richard Schwartz, PhD

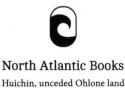

North Atlantic Books
Huichin, unceded Ohlone land
Berkeley, California

Published by
North Atlantic Books   Cover design by Howie Severson
Huichin, unceded Ohlone land   Book design by Happenstance Type-O-Rama
Berkeley, California   Printed in Canada

Somatic Internal Family Systems Therapy: Awareness, Breath, Resonance, Movement, and Touch in Practice is sponsored and published by North Atlantic Books, an educational nonprofit based in the unceded Ohlone land Huichin (Berkeley, CA) that collaborates with partners to develop cross-cultural perspectives; nurture holistic views of art, science, the humanities, and healing; and seed personal and global transformation by publishing work on the relationship of body, spirit, and nature.

North Atlantic Books's publications are distributed to the US trade and internationally by Penguin Random House Publisher Services. For further information, visit our website at www.northatlanticbooks.com.

Library of Congress Cataloging-in-Publication Data

Names: McConnell, Susan, 1948– author.
Title: Somatic internal family systems therapy : awareness, breath,
    resonance, movement and touch in practice / Susan McConnell ; foreword
    by Richard Schwartz, Ph.D.
Description: Berkeley, California : North Atlantic Books, [2020] | Summary:
    "Applying somatic principles to the Internal Family Systems model
    Somatic Internal Family Systems Therapy introduces a new therapeutic
    modality that blends principles of somatic therapy—like movement,
    touch, and breathwork—with the traditional tools of the Internal Family
    Systems framework. Broadening the benefits and applications of the IFS
    model, author Susan McConnell introduces 5 core practices that mental
    health professionals can apply to their practice: somatic awareness,
    conscious breathing, radical resonance, mindful movement, and attuned
    touch. Clinical applications include the treatment of depression,
    trauma, anxiety, eating disorders, chronic illness, and attachment
    disorders"— Provided by publisher.
Identifiers: LCCN 2020006693 | ISBN 9781623174880 (trade paperback)
Subjects: LCSH: Family psychotherapy. | Mind and body therapies. |
    Self-consciousness (Awareness) | Breathing exercises—Therapeutic use. |
    Movement therapy. | Touch—Therapeutic use.
Classification: LCC RC488.5 .M3918 2020 | DDC 616.89/156—dc23
LC record available at https://lccn.loc.gov/2020006693

7 8 9 10 11 MQ 26 25 24

Contents

Foreword

I AM VERY HONORED and excited that Susan McConnell has finally written this book that brings all of her wisdom from years of somatic study and practice to the Internal Family Systems (IFS) model, which I developed with lots of help from Susan along the way.

I remember those early years fondly. I had worked out the basics of IFS by the time Susan and I met around 1993, and she joined a small group of therapists I was leading in Chicago who were experimenting with our clients and each other to help me expand it and flesh it out. Those were exciting times and we all became very close to one another. While I am delighted with how IFS has now exploded in the US and around the world, I also long for those early days when we were more of a tight-knit little family searching for how to get it to where it is now.

Prior to meeting Susan, I had been collaborating with Ron Kurtz, the developer of Hakomi, a somatic- and mindfulness-based psychotherapy that complements IFS well. Ron and others in the Hakomi community had already influenced my approach to parts by making me aware of the importance of locating them in the body and directing communication with parts to those body locations. I also learned the value of sometimes letting a part take over and move one's body at times so that it felt fully witnessed.

Susan was a Hakomi trainer and a strong advocate for IFS to include even more somatic components, and now it does. She also became a leader in that growing IFS community. She was one of the first lead trainers and became a mentor to many of the subsequent ones (she was our first director of staff development). She had a passion for helping start things and was at my side for a lot of trainings, recording my talks and helping create experiential exercises with me on the fly. She was my trusted advisor through that time, and she produced the first training manual out of all that material she had been recording. For all of that I am eternally grateful.

She also had the courage to let me know when I was out of line. The parts of me that I leaned on to overcome my shyness and begin bringing IFS to a skeptical and sometimes hostile world of psychotherapy were not the parts best suited to leading a community. I needed someone to call me out when I was acting arrogant or thoughtless, and Susan and a few others often rose to that occasion. Because I trusted her and knew how much she cared for me and the future of IFS, I could hear it from her and I worked with those parts.

Over the years I have increasingly explored the relationship among what I call Self—the undamaged, healing essence within us all—parts, and the body. It is quite fascinating how parts can expel your Self from your body and how, when you are disembodied that way, it is more difficult for your Self to lead your system. So I have found the embodiment of Self to be an important goal in IFS. Self needs to be in the body to have enough purchase to be a good leader, and it is hard for parts to sense the comforting presence of Self when it is not embodied. When that is the case, parts, like parentless children, are in constant anxiety and become increasingly extreme. When Self is embodied, it is like the parent has returned home and the children can relax and be children.

No one has explored these issues more than Susan, and this book contains the practices she has discovered for achieving Self embodiment and for using the body to find parts and to heal them. As she has often said, we can only do violence to one another in this world if we are out of our body. So embodiment has implications for social activism and change.

IFS has become a big conceptual umbrella under which many approaches and perspectives fit well, as long as they have respect for the sacredness of parts and a belief in the existence of Self. I have been blessed over the years to have so many talented people bring their passions under this umbrella. (At last year's IFS conference I counted twenty-two such workshops—IFS EMDR, yoga, 12-step, meditation, breath work, anti-racism, constellation therapy, etc.) Somatic IFS tops the list of these valuable integrations, and I'm so grateful that Susan is giving us this extremely important gift.

—*Richard Schwartz, PhD, founder of Internal*
Family Systems therapy and the IFS Institute

Acknowledgments

ALTHOUGH WRITING FOR ME is a solitary act, throughout this experience I have felt the presence of countless people surrounding and supporting me. My most wholehearted appreciation goes to Beth O'Neil, my beloved spouse and life partner who has traveled with me, metaphorically and often literally, for four decades, sometimes accompanying and assisting me in my teaching all over the world, sometimes staying home to care for child, home, and pets, and, more recently, tolerating being abandoned to this book-writing project. Her wisdom and experience has influenced the development of Somatic IFS more than she imagines.

I give special thanks to Dick Schwartz, my friend and mentor, for believing in me. His tireless commitment to IFS has led to the expansion of the model all over the globe, to its inclusion as an evidence-based model of psychotherapy, and to it becoming a movement to bring Self energy to the world. From our earliest beginnings he has welcomed and affirmed my talents, including bringing the experiential and the somatic aspect more fully into IFS.

I am grateful for the many friends and teachers I have drawn from for my development of the practices of Somatic IFS, including Vickie Dodd, David Lauterstein, Alan Davidson, Jon Eisman, Ron Kurtz, Morgan Holford, Amina Knowlan, Bobby Rhodes, Susan Aposhyan, Deb Dana, Lisa Clark, and Cinda Rierson, who, on our frequent walks along Lake Michigan's shores, never failed to ask me how my book was coming. Kay Gardner has traveled with me from Hakomi to IFS trainer, laughing and crying along the way. The heart and hands of bodyworker Barry Krost have helped me reconnect with my bodymind system and my Embodied Self after injuries, illness, and negligence. Even as I write this acknowledgment, my dog reminds me to thank her for her ability to sense when I have been sitting at my computer for too long and for insisting that I stop tapping on my keyboard and play with her.

It never occurred to me to write a book on Somatic IFS until several people in the IFS community gently and repeatedly nudged me, even threatening to write it if I didn't. I want to thank Lois Ehrmann, Jennifer Baldwin, Mariel Pastor, Mary Steege, Susan Mason, and many other friends and colleagues and former students whose encouragement and book-writing and publishing experience buoyed me throughout the process. I am very grateful to North Atlantic Books for publishing my manuscript, and for my editor Gillian Hamel's gentle and respectful suggestions that improved this book and my writing skills. I am honored to have my book sit alongside their other publications that have profoundly influenced me throughout my career.

The core group of my Somatic IFS staff, Nancy Berkowitz, Fran Kolman, and Lois Ehrmann, have witnessed and influenced the emergence of Somatic IFS over the years, assisting many of our students in becoming more fully embodied in their Self energy. I feel a deep gratitude to them, and to the clients and the workshop, training, and retreat participants who have courageously shared their explorations into their bodymind systems. Their healing journeys have taught and inspired me, as I hope they will the readers.

Introduction

My Journey to Integrate Mind and Body

Including the body story along with the verbal story in therapy illuminates and awakens what has been obscured in darkness. The feral animal of our body, startled by the light, may scurry back to hide in the dark corners. The touch, the nourishment, the movement that our body craves may be buried under a history of neglect and trauma. We may feel our body has betrayed us. We may have internalized an objective attitude toward our body. Our individual hurts and collective societal burdens lodged in our tissues await the light of our courage and compassion shining into the depths of our interiority, leading us to the essence of our being.

As an Internal Family Systems (IFS) therapist and trainer I am committed to illuminating the somatic aspects of the inhabitants of the inner world of our psyches. I have developed Somatic IFS that consists of five practices that, when combined with the IFS model, work with the internal bodymind system to free up Embodied Self energy. This book begins with my journey that has placed me at the intersection of what Western culture has tried to keep separate, and it explores in depth the five practices of Somatic IFS that have been described as a branch of the tree of IFS. Not only have other IFS therapists been drawn to exploring the fruits from this branch, but also somatic therapists and educators, bodyworkers, and yoga practitioners, and anyone concerned with physical and emotional well-being. The practices of Somatic IFS—awareness, breathing, resonance, movement, and touch—provide a map for all of us who yearn for wholeness to enter safely into the rich territory of the bodymind.

I have traveled a work path with one foot in the world of the mind and another in the world of the body. My professional journey began with teaching children with physical disabilities—muscular dystrophy, cerebral palsy, spina bifida, and hearing and visual impairments—children whose movement limitations had affected their cognitive and emotional development. My entrance into the field of counseling began when the doors of the first domestic violence shelter in Chicago opened, as a parade of women sought refuge from abuse, each with a unique story of courage and defeat, many bringing their young, frozen-faced children. Listening to their stories of injury to body and mind, I hoped that the harboring household would allow the women to build a new life for themselves and their children. As I watched most of them return to their abusers, I was humbled by how little I understood about the crippling effects of physical and emotional trauma. I became overwhelmed by the complexity of the women's situations, the paperwork, and the staff infighting. When mysterious neuromuscular physical symptoms appeared in my body, at first I ignored them. The symptoms got worse. The various allopathic and alternative health practitioners I sought out did not provide a quick fix. In time I realized that what my body needed was a different relationship with me. Like the women at the shelter, I was caught in a passive, objectifying relationship with my body. My body could not be treated as if it were a car that could be taken in for maintenance and repair from overwork and neglect.

My shifting relationship with my body symptoms moved from fear and frustration to curious and tender regard. I slowed down. I listened. I stopped thinking so much. I became acquainted with the pulsations, the tones, and the vibrations of my tissues. I experimented. I found breath and movement practices that felt good to my body. My body movements and sensations led me to fears, grief, and anger. I shook and I sobbed. I began to understand how my perceptions, behaviors, and beliefs were shaping my body structure and function. Like the shelter residents, my physical and emotional scars were inseparable. Embracing them led to healing in both my mind and body. I came to understand that I *am* my body rather than I *have* a body.

It became clear that our culture had molded us to view our body from "the outside in." Digging into history, I learned that these cultural beliefs have been shaped by four hundred years of a dualistic view of mind and body that regards the mind and the soul as holy and exalted and the body as a subservient mortal carcass. It seemed like we were due for a paradigm shift.

Searching for resources that integrated mind and body, I finally found a book, now considered a classic, entitled *Bodymind*.[1] Not even a space between the words! I also learned about the philosopher and educator Thomas Hanna, who was pioneering the field of Somatics.[2] He coined the term "somatics" from the ancient Greek word *soma,* meaning body. Much of my learning and experimenting was convincing me that it is possible to overturn the mechanistic view of the body that has prevailed in Western cultures since the Enlightenment, that we could shed the objectification of our body as the Latin *corpus* and embrace this *soma,* this more subjective view of our body. We could view our body from the "inside out," honoring the body as a source of guidance and vessel for Spirit or life force. Changing ourselves can change the culture!

With the guidance of several teachers and masters I learned to listen to my insides—my bones, muscles, and viscera. Dance and other forms of movement such as martial arts and yoga, various kinds of bodywork, and other types of alternative healing all helped to return my body to a state of health. I decided to become a bodyworker to bring this form of healing to others.

Attending a bodywork class taught by Vickie Dodd, I discovered I was the only beginner in a class of the most advanced bodyworkers in Chicago. Vickie, knowing I was a potter as well as a counselor, reassured me that I could trust my hands that had learned to listen to clay and my heart that had learned to listen to the women at the shelter as I entered this new field. Instead of teaching us strokes or techniques, we learned about reciprocity. We discovered that when we tightened our jaws and our gluteal muscles as we touched our partner on the table, our partner's body resisted the touch. When we were grounded, centered, and relaxed, our partner's body opened to our touch and our hands were better able to listen to the skin and the underlying muscles and fascia.

My structural bodywork teachers taught me how to work with the connective tissue to increase my clients' awareness of their bodies' relationship to gravity and bring more coherence to their bodies. They emphasized the relationships between physical structure, function, and core beliefs. Shifts in the fascia often resulted in the release of the emotions. When the emotions weren't ready to be expressed, the fascia resisted the change.

Cranial sacral therapy offered a softer touch to integrate with the deep fascial work. As I listened with my hands to the subtle rhythmic waves of the cerebral spinal fluid, my clients became profoundly relaxed. Rather than making corrections to any abnormalities in the rhythms, I followed and mirrored them. I learned that attuning with the deeper tides at the core of the person accesses the inherent healing forces within their inner system. The body's innate intelligence restores the body's natural rhythms, affecting the brain, spinal cord, and autonomic nervous system. As the practitioner, I entered into a similar state as my client during the session and experienced a deep connection with my client that at times felt mystical.

Combining the earthy grounding of structural therapy and the watery realms of cranial sacral therapy was much like centering clay on my wheel as the water allowed the clay to take form. As I had with the clay, I was attuning to bodies to uncover the shapes wanting to be revealed. These two contrasting but complementary methods of bodywork brought many satisfying, sometimes profound, and lasting results—both physical and emotional. The clients who came to me had also reached a point in their lives where they could not keep ignoring the messages of their bodies. Their pain, like deeply rooted weeds that have been paved over, was finding the cracks and breaking through. The pain that had overwhelmed them was trapped in their bodies, and their symptoms, whether physical or mental or behavioral, were the pain's attempt to be heard and digested. As my clients spoke of the feelings and thoughts that arose when I touched into their tissues, I learned that the constricted places in the body's tissues and fluids held frozen feelings and memories. Many emotional releases were occurring on my bodywork table that seemed to correlate with the releases under my hands. As the body let go of what had been held for years, the mind did as well.

As much as I was learning about healing, I had even more questions. While my hands were exploring the tissues and witnessing the fluid rhythms with increasing skill and sensitivity, my mind was wondering how to help bring optimal relief and healing. How does change happen, and how can the changes "stick"? Is timing, the client's readiness to make a change, the primary factor? Will it be a technique—a stretch, a movement, or a particular kind of touch—that will open up the blocked areas, release the tension, and make a shift in the structure? Is it about manually freeing up fascia or sending energy? Or is the therapeutic relationship the primary agent of transformation? Is awareness the key? Is the cranial sacral therapy bypassing the client's awareness? Is my awareness alone enough, or is it important to include my client's awareness? Is the structural therapy invasive?

In addition to questions about healing the body, I could not disregard the emotional and cognitive aspects of my bodywork clients. Unfortunately, because of the prevalence of violence in our culture, most of my clients who wanted help with their bodies, especially my female clients, were carrying the scars of sexual, physical, and emotional abuse. Touching into the muscles, fascia, joints, and organs, I was aware I was touching into their trauma. The tissues might reveal the pain as my clients shared their stories in words and tears. Or their pain might be locked in the shortening and guarding of their myofascia or obstructions in the rhythmic flow of their energy. Often my clients were not able to be fully present to my touch.

At times I felt on shaky ground as I held in my awareness my clients' emotional life as well as their bodily experience. My approach was not supported by a culture where one looks to a therapist for help with one's feelings and thoughts and then to a bodywork practitioner for problems with the body. This cultural divorce of mind and body with its separate institutional regulatory agencies reinforces the internal splits most of us suffer from, whether they are due to conditioning, trauma, or both.

I found the guidance I needed for ways to integrate mind and body when the Hakomi training came to Chicago. This somatic psychotherapy method developed by Ron Kurtz is rooted in Buddhist mindfulness practices. Bringing awareness to what we are experiencing in the present moment in our body and our emotions gently and safely uncovers the core material that organizes our behavior, perceptions, and feelings. Awareness brings the possibility of choice. I learned experiential approaches to facilitate the transformation and reorganization of this core material. The ways we move and hold ourselves reveal and allow for a direct dialogue with our implicitly held beliefs and emotions. I learned to listen to the gestures, pace, posture, voice quality, changes in energy, and breathing patterns as well as the spoken words. The principles of the Hakomi method became foundational in my life and my work. I became a teacher of Hakomi. I learned more about working with trauma through the body by studying with then-Hakomi trainer Pat Ogden, who went on to develop Sensorimotor Psychotherapy. I incorporated and adapted the principles and methods of Hakomi into my bodywork practice, and I developed and taught a training in Hakomi for bodyworkers.

The mindful approach of Hakomi led me to Buddhism to deepen my mindfulness practice. Zen Buddhism increased my awareness of my body sensations and my inner world. Although the body in Buddhism can be ignored and denied to a similar degree as in other religions, mindfulness practice as taught by the Buddha includes the body. One of my favorite stories about the Buddha is when on the verge of enlightenment and confronted about his authority to claim enlightenment, his response was to reach out with his right hand to touch the earth. I can imagine how utterly present he was in his body as he sat on the earth. His awareness was more powerful than an eloquent exegesis or persuasive defense. With that gesture, his final obstacle to enlightenment dissolved and Siddhartha became the Buddha, the Awakened One.

Zen master Bobby Rhodes, a.k.a. Soeng Hyang of the Kwan Um School of Zen, became my teacher. Sitting in silence for days at a time, I could not avoid the sensations of numbness and pain in my legs and back and the parade of judgments and criticisms flooding my mind. My mental and physical obstacles eventually dissolved, leaving me feeling surprisingly connected with the other people sitting with me in silence. At each interview Bobby would present me with a koan, a puzzling paradoxical story or situation that requires a response. I was expected to respond to the question by hitting the floor and saying, "Don't know." This action stopped my mind from trying to figure out the right answer. The smacking of my hand on the floor and the words cutting through the conditioning from years of schooling would help me to enter into the heart of the koan, allowing a more intuitive response to emerge. As with the story of the Buddha's enlightenment, the answers to the koans often took the form of a body movement or gesture that expressed the nature of my immediate personal relationship with the presented situation.

During these years while I was exploring, learning, teaching, and engaged in healing myself and others, Richard Schwartz was engaged in getting his PhD in marriage and family therapy, attaining the status of associate professor at both the University of Illinois and Northwestern University, and writing a family-therapy text. As he listened with an open heart, a curious mind, and the ear of a trained structural family therapist to his clients' descriptions of their inner struggles and conflicts, he conceptualized their inner worlds in ways similar to how he viewed the interrelationships in the family. He heard clients speak of a "part" of them that had emotions, perceptions, and belief systems.

As Schwartz listened to these aspects of their psyches, they seemed much more than pale disembodied interjects, rarified archetypes, or internalized representations of external figures. When these subpersonalities felt seen, heard, and related to as if they were individuals, they let him know they had been longing to be seen and heard. As he listened to his clients' descriptions of their inner worlds, he realized that these parts reveal the range of emotions, histories, purposes, perspectives, beliefs, and behaviors as do actual people. They most often appear as young people, of any gender, independent of the client's gender.

This concept of multiplicity of the personality is not new, to either psychotherapy models, poets, or politicians. But Schwartz added a system aspect to his developing model as he learned that these parts had relationships with other parts in the client's system that were as complex as relationships in any family. The parts might be protective and critical, dependent and rebellious, or caretaking and resentful. Approaching these parts in the same way he approached the members of a family, he found their behaviors eventually became less extreme and their interrelationships more collaborative. His clients often experienced a profound resolution of the symptoms that had brought them into therapy.

One more crucial piece of his model was incorporated as the parts relaxed in the atmosphere of safety and respect, making space for another aspect of his clients' personalities to be freed up. Schwartz's clients described this state as distinct from any of the parts they had discovered—a state that has the wisdom and compassion they had previously attributed to him. His clients referred to this state not as a part but simply as "my Self," so he adopted this word for this core essence in each person. As he developed his unique approach to therapy through his work, his study, and his writing, he adopted his clients' terminology of "parts" and "Self" and came to call his model Internal Family Systems, or IFS.

If the concept of multiplicity of the personality is challenging to some, the assumption that *everyone* has a Self is a fairly radical notion. At the core of every individual, when all the extra is peeled away, is this essential loving, creative, wise, courageous state. This assumption is itself an intervention in therapy. It changes the role of the therapist from the interpreter, analyzer, or problem solver to the one who uncovers this essential Self in their client. The Self energy of the therapist and client is the agent of transformation. The goal of IFS therapy came to be the liberation of this inherent state to its rightful place of leadership by befriending isolated, distressed, and untrusting parts that were obscuring this inherent goodness and wisdom. When parts' trust in the Self is restored, all the parts of the system can be helped to let go of their extreme, survival-oriented roles and reorganize in collaborative and harmonious relationships. Once a client's Self is available in the inner system, the client no longer depends solely on the therapist's Self.

Schwartz likens the noncoercive, collaborative style of leadership of Self to that of a good orchestra conductor. At times playing an observing, witnessing role, and at others an active compassionate presence, Self energy is similar to how light photons can manifest as both particles and waves. He describes both aspects of Self: "As an entity, it is available to hear competing perspectives, to nurture, and to problem-solve. As a wave, it is one with the universe and other people as if, at that level, all waves overlap in ultimate commonality."[3] He increasingly saw his job was to get out of the way when the client's Self had emerged and to support it as the agent of healing in the client's system. With the exponential power of Self in the therapy room, the client's healing takes a quantum leap.

In a recent conference plenary I participated in with IFS therapist Jan Mullen, Jan shared her reflections on the early days of IFS: "The IFS model came on the scene when therapy was reliant on the cognitive analysis of the therapist, based on theories such as psychoanalytic and self psychology, and has been on the cutting edge of a more wholistic, directly experiential therapy. It was an uphill climb to challenge the prevailing monolithic view of the person and assert the natural multiplicity of the human mind."

Although Schwartz is a rather quiet, unassuming man, his passion for his model was contagious. Like a magnet he drew toward him like-minded people who were intrigued with his model and eager to find a way to contribute to the development of IFS. As Schwartz was living near Chicago and was finding some resonance between IFS and Hakomi, eventually our paths coincided. I could not have foreseen that this connection would reshape my professional life for (as of this writing) the next twenty-five years. I was initially drawn to his earnestness, humility, openness, and his commitment to his own healing. I particularly valued that he had the courage to put his structural family therapy training on a shelf and allow his emerging model to arise from listening to his clients. Schwartz is called Dick by his friends and colleagues, and I was honored to become among them. The IFS model and organization were shaped in those early days by a few people sitting on the floor of my office who had been drawn to Dick and this new approach.

It was my need for consultation rather than a search for a new therapy model that launched me on this life-changing path. I had been having substantial results with Hakomi and I enjoyed teaching the model to both the psychotherapeutic and the bodywork communities. I joined Dick's consultation group when a client of mine nearly succeeded at killing herself with an overdose. In addition to supporting me, the consultation group gave me the opportunity to learn his developing approach to therapy.

In this group I learned that some of our parts hold the painful emotions of our abandonment or trauma, referred to as "exiles," while others are forced into protecting these vulnerable parts or protecting the system from further hurts. The protective parts called "managers" exhibit various behaviors such as critical, controlling strategies, while the ones referred to as "fire-fighters" react impulsively when the vulnerable feelings threaten to arise. Most all of these parts are much younger than one's chronological age. This internal family of parts adopts oppositional strategies with each other that lock the system into rigid dysfunctional relationships. The protectors are overworked, isolated, besieged, and beleaguered. The vulnerable ones are typically exiled. They are desperate, lonely, and needy. They continue to get wounded externally as well as internally by the parts that are attempting to protect them. The inner system is caught in a proverbial Catch-22. The protectors cannot abandon their posts until the vulnerable ones are safely cared for, but the vulnerable ones can't be cared for until the protectors relax their grip.

Being an IFS therapist is a bit like being an archeologist sifting through the layers of ancient remains and discovering how they fit together and the histories they reveal. Who are these parts? What do they do? How long have they been doing/feeling/believing this? Are they friends or enemies? Do they form gangs, do they hide out, dominate, protect? My job was to help the client find these parts and unearth their own Self energy buried under the burdened parts.

IFS offered a compassionate view of my clients' protector parts. Whether they are being critical, controlling, rageful, manipulative, or simply inauthentic, the protectors can be hard to cozy up to. Parts that "resist" therapy are the bane of the therapy world, and the "borderline" label causes many of us to flinch. Although their behaviors result in often catastrophic and heart-rending consequences, I came to understand that these protector parts were forced into extreme roles, usually at a very young age. Despite the fact that their behaviors lead to quite tragic outcomes—ironically often the very outcome they had been trying to prevent—they all mean well. Their detrimental actions are based on their distorted perceptions, which in turn are colored by the burdens and pressures within their internal and external systems. The protectors believe it's all up to them to hold down the fort. Nearly all my clients have been hurt in their early lives to such an extent that their protectors are diligent in the extreme. I now understood my clients' self-destructive acts were behaviors of these young, misguided but well-intentioned parts. These valiant protectors will only truly transform once they are assured the ones they are protecting are safe—safe from within and from without.

At birth Self energy, though inherently present, has not yet developed the physical, neurological, or experiential capacity to either prevent the hurt or to heal it. In some cases, Self energy was pushed out of the system for its own protection, like a ruler driven into exile until order is restored. But this core essential Self now has clarity, courage, wisdom, and confidence, and the protectors actually long to let go of their burdened roles. It is common for clients to first rely on the Self energy of the therapist until their parts feel more trusting. Sensing Self energy—of the therapist and/or the client—the client's protectors share why they did what they did, and even what they would rather do if only that were possible.

As the protectors share their side of the story, the vulnerable parts they were protecting are revealed. These young parts are desperately and tragically looking everywhere for reassurance and redemption but to the only truly dependable source—the Self. Like young children with their noses pressed to the window looking for a savior, they simply need to turn around to see their savior is in the room with them. They can be retrieved from where and when they were frozen or imprisoned. They find safety and healing in their relationship with Self. As their suppressed stories are heard, they are ready to let go of the burdens—the emotions, sensations, thoughts, and behaviors—they accumulated from their injuries. They often find a creative way of releasing their burdens—sending them to the light, burying them deep in the earth, hurling them over a cliff, or dissolving them in a sacred pool. The burden is gone while the part remains, restored to its inherent role in the system.

The ecology of our inner systems is such that as even one part is able to trust Self energy enough to let go of the limiting beliefs that had distorted its roles, other parts in the internal system are also able to make a shift. The furniture of our inner room can rearrange into a more comfortable and harmonious pattern. Parts that had been trying to protect the part from further harm, parts that had been trying to maintain some semblance of balance in the system, realize they can finally relax their decades-long efforts. They remember or rediscover or sometimes create their preferred roles. Parentified managers are able to rest in the security of knowing Self is in the lead. Dissociating or impulsive, reactive firefighters can become playful and creative. I glimpsed the path to make it possible for all the parts to become connected with Self and with each other in harmonious, collaborative relationships.

I came to personally know the power of this model when I shared about my suicidal client in the consultation group. I had expected Dick to instruct me in how to apply this model in this situation. Instead, he asked me to look and listen inside to see what was coming up within me. Tuning in to my body, my images, thoughts, and feelings, I found a protector that criticized me for having failed my client, and another one that was casting about for some way to make sure my client would not attempt to end her life again. My vulnerable parts held fear and powerlessness. Dick coached me to listen respectfully and appreciatively to these parts. I realized these parts were young—too young to be taking over my therapist chair and trying to help this young woman. They were more than happy to allow me to take back my seat.

When I next saw my client I was able to listen deeply and calmly to the parts of her that wanted to end her life. I had known that she had been her alcoholic mother's caregiver until her mother's death, when at the age of eight she was raised by her older sister and her sister's husband who groomed her to be his "mistress." When she told her family about this abuse they turned against her, blaming and shunning her. Her suicidal part saw death as the only path to end her suffering. When instead of trying to manage her suicidal part I brought compassion to it, the part was open to considering there could be another way to lessen her pain. This made space to hear from her parts that did not want her to die, as well as the ones that held numerous burdens from the sexual abuse.

Integrating IFS into my therapeutic work was fairly seamless. The model made intuitive and intellectual sense to me. Many of my clients were mindfully exploring their inner worlds. Some of them were already using the word "part" since this is fairly common parlance. One client said with relief, "I'm not the angry vicious monster I thought I was. I just have a part that is angry." He said it was like his part had embedded within him an angry virus, like a computer virus. The tough things in his life had corrupted his young part's innocence, and this virus was like malware that altered his behavior. He was relieved to hear we could remove the virus and restore his inner operating system.

IFS was providing me with another vehicle for my own healing as well as helping me become a more compassionate therapist. Faced with a client in the throes of some extreme behavior or emotion, I could remember that Self energy, when not evident, is simply blanketed like the sun on a cloudy day, and my distancing parts, over-empathizing parts, and rescuing or caretaker parts relaxed. I shifted my responsibility from being the source of my clients' healing to trying to stay in Self energy so I could help my clients uncover theirs. I became solidly grounded in the IFS model even as I continued to draw from my bodywork and Hakomi background. Integrating these models helped me shepherd my clients through their profound personal journeys, working with my own parts—and those of the client—to prepare a welcoming environment for Self leadership.

Shortly after his first book, *Internal Family Systems Therapy*,[4] came out, Dick encouraged me to participate in the training soon to begin in Chicago. I hadn't decided to take the training until a dream determined my future. In the dream I was sitting at a long table with some Hakomi colleagues at one end and Dick at the other. In the dream I approached him, remembering I had wanted to ask him about the upcoming Chicago IFS training. He responded by telling me there were two trainings—one had about thirty people in it, and it was already full. The other had four, and this smaller one was the one he wanted me to be in. With that, the music began to play and Dick and I began to dance. I was leading. He gave me a huge smile and said to me, "I like not having to lead all the time." When I shared the dream with Dick, he told me he understood what the group of four meant. He explained to me that his plan for the training was to lead the whole group for all but the last two hours of the day when four assistants would lead small groups, demonstrating the model, leading experiential exercises and discussions. "I can do that!" I responded. "OK, you're in," he said. We laughed together as he also admitted to me that in dancing with his wife he liked not having to lead all the time.

Before long I came to understand how prophetic was the ending of the dream. This model was really catching on! Beyond our nation's heartland, therapists from both coasts were asking for IFS trainings. It soon became obvious that Dick could not train all the people who were eager to learn IFS. I began in earnest to document his talks about his model along with the experiential components I and other assistants had been developing to complement the didactic elements. I realized that others of us would soon be needed to step up to lead trainings. From this dream, and my willingness to lead the dance, I developed a training curriculum for students and trainers based, in part, on what I had recorded. In this first IFS training manual, I wove into the curriculum a more experiential and body-based approach to the trainings.

This more body-centered approach began to emerge out of exile and seep back into my work with clients. The whisper of the potential power of including the body more fully into every step of the model lurked at the edges of my imagination. Like something waiting in the darkness to be birthed, the somatic approach needed me to breathe into it and occasionally push it toward the light. I connected *what* my clients were saying to *how* they were saying it. I began to linger with the sensations they were experiencing. The sensations were at the core. The words, images, and emotions sprung from the sensations. Staying with the physical sensations and following where they led us revealed the stories behind or alongside the verbal words—the body stories. We began to in*corp*orate them with the verbal stories. I reclaimed that, for me, psychotherapy is physiology. Engaging with my clients in the process of psychotherapy is delving into a somatic state of relatedness no less physiological than breathing, birthing, and dying. I could not listen with my ears alone. I listened with my eyes tracking my clients' gestures, posture, facial expressions, and movement. I listened with my body—and to my body—noticing tensions, flowing energy, prickles, trembles, warmth, heaviness, and shifts in the breath. I listened with my hands with clients who were open to physical contact. Information about my clients' inner worlds was flowing into me through my eyes, my body, and my hands.

Dick was open to a more body-centered approach to therapy. Although he admitted his awareness of his body was mostly limited to its use on the football field or the basketball court, he recognized the value of including the body in working with the internal family. IFS includes the body in a couple steps of the process. For example, when the client identifies a part, regardless of whether it appears as a thought, an emotion, or an image, we ask the client where they feel it in their body. We also may locate the burdened emotion or belief in the body. The IFS model as we have taught it in the United States and internationally is not incomplete or lacking in effectiveness without a more expansive body component. It has earned its status as an evidence-based model. I have been honored to teach the model and to contribute to its evolution over the years. It is as if IFS has been absorbed into the marrow of my bones and is dissolved in all my bodily fluids.

My IFS students sensed there was something different in my approach to IFS as they watched me work. They described it as a more "feminine" approach—more right-brained, still structured, but less linear, in some ways more relational, more intuitive. Many of them felt congruence with this way of working and asked for more training. Many clients, students, and therapists were interested in bringing the body more fully into IFS. Some of them had been steeped in somatic practices in their lives, like through yoga, dance, and bodywork. Others processed primarily kinesthetically. Many had studied body-centered approaches like Somatic Experiencing, Hakomi, Sensorimotor Psychotherapy. They looked to Somatic IFS for help synthesizing these valuable approaches with IFS, or perhaps they had only a basic understanding of IFS to integrate into these modalities. Others felt that they had parts that have exiled their physicality because of trauma or cultural and religious influences. They said that they are "too much in their heads" and wanted support and training to correct that imbalance. These people had approached me to explore what benefits might occur from bringing the body more fully into the IFS model.

My experience has convinced me that every therapeutic issue can benefit from integrating the somatic aspect of our internal system. The body-based interventions help us in the places where we get stuck. Somatic IFS emphasizes that Self must be embodied for its fullest expression. It provides a path for that. As individuals free their Embodied Selves, the transformation ripples outward to affect the various institutions of our culture that have been influenced by four hundred years of separation of mind and body. Perhaps it can counteract societal forces that have truncated our capacity for embodiment, such as religious institutions that devalue and even demonize the body, and schools that require little children to sit and walk quietly in rows for hours at a time, and our consumerist and media-driven culture that distracts us from our body awareness. Somatic IFS joins many other body-mind approaches as an antidote to those cultural influences.

Inspired by Dick Schwartz's process of developing IFS through listening to his clients, Somatic IFS has developed from listening to my body and my clients' bodies as we explore our inner systems.[5] My development of Somatic IFS also has been nourished by the work of the many pioneers in the field of body-centered psychotherapies as well as somatic practices that have helped me uncover and sustain Embodied Self energy. Rather than creating a separate model, what emerged from my studies and experience is a branch of this sturdy and expanding tree, or, as others have suggested, a hybrid tree, growing in the same field. I call this branch (or this tree) "Somatic IFS," rooted in the same assumptions of multiplicity and drawing from the transformative energy of Self.

Through teaching this synthesis of various methods, models, and approaches, I have focused on five core interdependent practices that, integrated into the IFS model, lead to a state of Embodied Self. Each of these practices will be described and explored in depth in this book. The foundational practice is **Somatic Awareness.** Awareness of the body naturally leads to the practice of **Conscious Breathing.** Breath is the bridge to the relational realm with the practice of **Radical Resonance.** With the practice of **Mindful Movement** we bring awareness to spontaneous movements and initiate specific movements to facilitate each step of the model. All the practices support **Attuned Touch.** offering a safe, and often neglected, communication pathway between parts and Self.

The structure of the book could be compared to the organization of the body. If the IFS model is the skeleton of Somatic IFS, providing the scaffolding for the practices, the five practices could be viewed as separate but interrelated systems of the body attached to the bones. Just as the flesh, viscera, nervous system, and circulatory system are considered as separate body systems yet understood to function as interrelated and interdependent aspects of the body, each of the five practices of Somatic IFS function similarly.

The first chapter provides an overall view of Somatic IFS and illustrates how a somatic approach can integrate into every step of the IFS model. Subsequent chapters explore each of the practices of Somatic IFS. Delving into each of the practices in depth provides the reader with a growing understanding of how to incorporate somatic practices into their clinical and professional work. Exercises and case studies are woven throughout the theoretical aspects of each practice to provide experiential and clinical applications. Specific body systems are associated with each practice as a path to helping the reader embody the conceptual material and to appreciate the systemic nature of the bodymind. Somatic IFS, while benefitting from recent scientific research, also draws from many healing and religious traditions. Each practice is associated with a classical element. Incorporating earth, air, water, and fire in the exploration of each practice ties Somatic IFS to these traditions and links the human organism—mind, body, and spirit—with the cosmic body made up of these elements.

As Somatic IFS invites the body from its exiled state as *corpus* to a living, breathing, transformative entity, we work with the body as carefully as with any exile. We assess if the external reality is truly safe enough to permit a return to embodiment. As we work with our own parts as well as those of the clients, we prepare a welcoming environment for the somatic aspect of our internal systems. My hope is that my lifetime exploration of mind and body healing practices that has culminated in this book can be an invitation and a guide for others on a similar healing path. I have found that these somatic practices have facilitated my work with clients with every therapeutic issue, including chronic illness, addictions, trauma, attachment wounds, and sexual and relational issues. My clients have transformed their bodies and their relationships with their bodies and with others. Somatic IFS owes a deep gratitude to both the IFS model and pioneers in the field of body-centered psychotherapies.

The irony does not escape me that I am endeavoring to craft the words to bring to life that which is often wordless, that which when attempted to make verbal or explain or describe may cause it to scurry away to hide again in the dark corners. I have learned that I need to use these Somatic IFS practices as I sit for hours at my computer, typing and gazing at my monitor. When my back started complaining greatly, I turned again to Thomas Hanna's book *Somatics*. The exercises eventually helped restore my body's health and ease. I frequently lie on the floor and go inside to experience what I am writing about, and to write about what I am experiencing. I invite you to try out the ideas and the practices presented in this book to discover how they work for you and your clients.

This book is a guide for anyone working at the interface of body and mind who wants to be in a healthy and healing relationship with others. I hope that the ideas and practical potentials embedded in this book will lead to the profound changes needed at every level of system. The next chapter provides an in-depth introduction to Somatic IFS.

1

Introduction to Somatic IFS
and the Practices That
Lead to Embodied Self

IN THE EARLY 1900s, a very special horse named Clever Hans astonished the public with his intelligence. He could perform all kinds of mathematical calculations, tell time, read, spell, and understand German. He correctly answered questions by tapping his hoof. A special Hans Commission was convened to explore this phenomenon. The scientists eventually realized that Hans was responding to the unconsciously transmitted nonverbal cues from the questioner—his movements, tensions, and facial expressions. Clever Hans was not as clever with math as was first assumed, but his unusual sensitivities helped researchers understand the bias that comes from unconscious cueing in non-double-blind tests.

What allowed this particular horse to be able to pick up on his owner's nonverbal cues? Did he have a particularly resonant relationship with his owner that sharpened his sensory awareness of his owner's facial expressions, body tensions, subtle changes in his breathing or movement? Was the sense of touch involved? Did the owner unknowingly transmit the correct answer through some subtle change in his holding of the bridle?

Since this horse awed the public there have been animals of other species that for some reason demonstrated exceptional abilities to communicate with humans. Their stories remind us of the innate ability we share with other animals to receive vast amounts of information transmitted nonverbally and mostly unconsciously. Our hunter-gatherer ancestors' lives depended on this ability and used it solely before spoken language evolved. Today we rely far more on *what* is being said than *how* it is being said.

The Five Practices of Somatic IFS

Somatic IFS therapists hone their sensitivities and enhance their "horse sense" with somatic practices, all in service of their clients' healing. Opening to a deep, heartfelt connection with their clients, they listen to how their clients are saying what they are saying. They attend to slight shifts in voice quality, facial expressions, and muscular tone. They are conscious of their clients' breathing and of their involuntary movements. If touch is an aspect of the relationship, even a handshake or a hug, they listen to the information being transmitted through that touch as well.

The Somatic IFS therapist develops the practices of Somatic Awareness, Conscious Breathing, Radical Resonance, Mindful Movement, and Attuned Touch and brings these practices to every step of the IFS model. In subsequent chapters each of these practices will be explored in detail with examples of how the practices are integrated into IFS. These practices are to some degree sequential, depending on the previous practice for a fuller experience of the subsequent one. They are also interdependent. For example, Conscious Breathing depends on Somatic Awareness since one cannot be conscious of their breathing without awareness. Conscious Breathing relies on awareness and can also enhance one's facility with the practice of Somatic Awareness. Resonance depends on awareness, is facilitated by breath, and can mirror movements or use touch to enhance resonance. In this book we will explore how each practice and all of them in total lead to the experience of Embodied Self energy and how they all require some degree of Embodied Self energy to engage in the practice.

While our clients' words are important, their postures, movements, and voice tones are impacting us, and ours are impacting them. We are affecting each other through our body language in myriad and largely unconscious ways. As we attend to the language of the body, we increase our awareness of the 70 percent of communication that is nonverbal happening in our therapy rooms. Simply put, these five practices of Somatic IFS that are the substance of this book develop and retrain our attentional sensory habits and help us become as exceptional a therapist as Clever Hans was a horse.

Somatic IFS has emerged in large part because of the many therapists and practitioners who are looking to bridge the chasm between body and mind in the field of psychotherapy. While the body is included to some extent in IFS trainings, the intention of Somatic IFS is to include the body and the somatic practices in every step of the therapeutic process to work with every clinical issue. Not only do we incorporate somatic practices with every step of IFS, we deepen and expand our awareness of how the body is participating in each step. The powerful and empowering IFS model becomes more three-dimensional—a cognitive, emotional, spiritual, and physiological process that lives and breathes. As Dick Schwartz has quoted me in his latest edition of *Internal Family Systems Therapy:*

> As parts absorb burdens over the course of a lifetime, the body's awareness, breathing patterns, ability to resonate with others, to move with ease, grace, and freedom, and to give and receive touch are all adversely affected, [but] psychic as well as physical injury that occurs in the body . . . can be healed in the body.[1]

Somatic IFS incorporates the five practices to heal parts' burdens in the body, using the IFS model. In teaching IFS we have found it helpful to describe the process of the therapy in sequential steps. Using an example from a session with my client Tim, we can see how Somatic IFS integrates into each step of the IFS model.

The Steps of Somatic IFS

The Therapist Assesses the External Situation of the Client

The first step is for the therapist to assess whether the client's external situation allows them to engage in a process of inner work. The client's safety often comes down to basic physical needs of their body. Do they have food, shelter, and adequate medical care? Are they safe from physical harm? Does the client have adequate social resources to support inner work? If not, the therapist first attends to these basic needs and stabilizes the client's external physical environment.

> Tim enters my office for his first session. The shoulders of his sport coat are hiked up around his ears. He plops down in the chair across from me, looks at his hands, and rubs his fingers together. I recall that he told me on the phone that he recently left his successful professional career in the corporate world and is finding odd jobs to supplement his severance pay while he considers his next steps, so it seems that there are no obvious external constraints affecting our work together. Tim does not appear to feel safe, but I am guessing this has more to do with what is happening inside of him.

The Therapist Embodies Self Energy

Being in the therapist role can bring up our vulnerable parts. Although the therapist holds more power in a therapeutic relationship and the client is in the more vulnerable position, we therapists may have fearful parts, especially with a new client or a challenging client. We find the fears in our body. Rather than *trying* to relax, adding a layer of parts onto the tense part, we start with noticing the tension. Then we bring a quick moment of compassion and reassurance to the fearful part. The tension lets go enough for us to find a place in our body to draw from—our spine or our heart, or any place that feels open to connecting with the client across from us.

> I notice the sensations of the weight of my shoes on the floor. I breathe in and out as I lengthen my spine while I look at Tim. I feel a slight collapse in the upper part of my chest. My heart is beating faster than usual. I breathe in and out a few more times, filling up the empty space in my chest. I bring my energy back down into my belly. I begin to feel a bit more relaxed and centered. During these few seconds, I've been noticing Tim's eyes dart around the room. I'm curious about that and eager to learn more about how he is doing.

The Therapist Attends to the Client's Safety in the Therapy Office

Once the therapist knows the client is physically safe in their home environment, the therapist then attends to the client's safety in the therapy office. How is the physical space of the office perceived by the client? As much as possible, the therapist attends to the client's needs for a shift in room furniture, air temperature, lighting, and any objects that may interfere with a sense of being safely held in the physical environment.

> I ask Tim to check in to see how the distance between us feels to him. He moves his chair further and further away until it is in the furthest corner of the room. Many of my clients may shift the chair a few inches one way or the other, but Tim is the first one to choose to sit so far away. I am surprised and curious. I wonder if I should be alarmed. But then Tim lets out a big sigh.
>
> Tim: You know, I've never had someone ask me about this before, to be that concerned that I feel safe here.
>
> I feel my whole body relax. I smile at Tim.

The Therapist Contracts with the Client

The therapist and client get agreement on how to work together and what to work on. The Somatic IFS therapist listens to the verbal as well as the non-verbal communication. Concerning this contract step, the therapist is listening for incongruences between what the client is saying and how they are saying it. The contract may need to change over time. When I am offering supervision to IFS therapists, this step is often at the root of the difficulties.

> Tim tells me he wants to limit his alcohol consumption. He had been drinking because of the stress at work, but even now after several weeks of not working, he is finding he is drinking even more. With these words, he looks away and his voice drops.
>
> SM: We can definitely work with your drinking behavior, but first I want to know if you have any hesitations, any concerns, about limiting your drinking.
> Tim: Well, I have tried to do this before, both limiting it and stopping, and it hasn't worked too well. I'm afraid to try again. I'll probably fail again.
> SM: I'd like to first work with this part in order to clear the path to work with the drinking. How does that sound?
>
> Tim looks in my eyes for a moment, and then he nods. I notice he didn't object to my using the word "part."

The Therapist Works with the Protector Parts with "the Six Fs"

When we teach the IFS model, we offer six steps to working with protector parts so they will trust the Self to work with the vulnerable exiles. We identify words that include the letter F in each step as a mnemonic device. The first three steps involve helping the client see that the part's feelings and beliefs are separate from their own self: **F**ind the part, **F**ocus on it, and **F**lesh it out. The last three steps help establish an Embodied Self-to-part relationship: ask the client how they **F**eel toward the part, be**F**riend the part, and address the part's Fears. These six steps are not a strict formula and are not necessarily sequential. They are helpful for the therapist to guide the session along.

Somatic IFS uses these same six steps to guide the flow of the process, with some modifications. Our case example with Tim illustrates each of these steps in Somatic IFS through the lens of the six Fs. Later chapters will make more explicit how somatic awareness, breath, resonance, movement, and touch can facilitate these steps.

1. FINDING THE PART

The IFS therapist is trained to ask, "Where do you find this part in or around your body?" Ironically the Somatic IFS therapist does not ask this question. We do not assume the client can initially find the part in or around their body. The client may hear the part speaking to him, or he may speak from the part. He may see the part as himself, or a younger version of himself. He may see a particular memory of an earlier experience. He may have thoughts that are clearly coming from the part or are thoughts about the part coming from another part. He may show behaviors that are expressions of the part. He may be aware of an emotion and label it but not be aware of it in his body. He may have only the vaguest sense of what we are referring to as a part, yet this vagueness is enough for him to begin to experience the difference between himself and this other part of him.

The Somatic IFS therapist is noting how the part first shows up in the client's experience. However the client responds, the therapist brings awareness to their own somatic experience as well as the client's nonverbal communication to help the client turn their attention inward to connect with the part, however it makes its first appearance.

SM: Tim, can you find the part that you just named that is afraid to try to limit your drinking because it hasn't worked out so well in the past?

Tim doesn't initially turn his attention inward. He stays outwardly focused on me. He tells me about his past drinking and goes into some detail about his past failed attempts to limit his drinking. I'm listening to his words and watching his body and mine as well. He is sitting up straighter in his chair and his neck looks stiffly held. My neck feels a little stiff too, and my lumbar area is tightening. I breathe in and out and bring my navel toward my belly on my exhale. I wonder what can help him turn his attention inside. Although the second F step is usually "focusing on the part," I am not sure that focusing on the explaining part, or asking him to focus on his bodily tension, will engage his curiosity. I decide to skip to "fleshing out the part." Perhaps piquing his curiosity will help him go inside.

2. FLESHING OUT THE PART

"Fleshing out" means to get to know more than one aspect of a part. However a part first appears, it is only once we know the part as more than a sensation or more than a feeling that this subpersonality takes on the impression of being a part we can relate to as a person with a history, behaviors, hopes. The therapist invites the part to be known as fully as possible by asking questions, or coaching the client's Self to ask questions of the part. The Somatic IFS therapist is aware of integrating "top down" and "bottom up" processing while the thoughts and beliefs of the part are held in awareness, along with sensations and movement impulses.

I am thinking I may be able to engage Tim's curiosity about his part that has trepidations about his stated therapeutic goal as a first step toward going inside. Maybe once we have a sense of the physical sensations of the part, Tim will find it easier to focus on the part.

SM: Tim, I want to hear more about your drinking, but let's first get to better know this part that doesn't want to try again so we know how to help it. Can you notice what is happening in your body as you are telling me this?

Tim looks at me in surprise, closes his eyes, lifts his chin, and looks again at me.

Tim: I guess I feel a little nervous.

3. FOCUSING ON THE PART

This step begins the process of differentiating the part from Self by establishing a relationship with the part. To help the client keep their attention focused on the part, we may ask questions about the part's location, the qualities of the sensations connected with the part, and how those sensations change over time.

I haven't heard what is happening in his body, but Tim's answer has fleshed the part out to include an emotion. Because emotions are inseparable from our body sensations, I ask Tim to focus on the nervous feeling. He closes his eyes and is quiet.

SM: What in your body lets you know you are nervous?
Tim: [*touching his stomach*] I guess it's in my gut.
SM: Would it be OK to just stay with the sensations in your gut?
Tim: It's pretty tight in there . . . it's even tighter up here. [*touching the area of his diaphragm*]
SM: Does it have a weight, or is the tension pulling?
Tim: It's pulling.
SM: Can you tell what direction it's pulling?
Tim: Yes, it is pulling upward. It's getting tighter. [*His chest lifts up and his breathing is shallow.*]
SM: It looks like this is uncomfortable. Is it OK so far?
Tim: Yeah, it's OK.

FLESHING OUT THE PART (AGAIN)

Repeating this step shows that the IFS process in practice is not always linear, but it is a guide to working effectively and safely with the internal system rather than an exact formula.

SM: As you hold your stomach, ask this part in your stomach if it has words or an image that go with this tight feeling.
Tim: I don't know if this is connected, but I am remembering being a teenager. I see him in my bedroom when we lived in Westville.

> SM: Ask the nervous part if it is showing you this memory to let you know the teenager is feeling nervous.
> Tim: The part says yes.
>
> By now Tim has a fuller sense of this part—it is nervous, it shows up as tension in his stomach and as an image of himself as a teenager. The teenager has a behavior (isolating in his room) and this teenager is anxious.
>
> SM: Can he tell you or show you what he is nervous about?
> Tim: He is scared of his dad. He is also sick of being controlled, not being trusted, not being able to do what he wants to do.
>
> Tim's part is ready to be addressed in its fullness from Embodied Self energy. Either Tim's or mine. The next step will reveal if Tim's Self energy is present.

4. ASKING HOW THE CLIENT FEELS TOWARD THE PART

The fourth F continues differentiating the part from Self energy by asking the client how they feel toward the part. In IFS the primary agent of healing is between the client's Self and their part. A relationship between these two states is facilitated by the therapist. It requires that the part has not completely dominated the client's system—a situation we refer to in IFS as the part has "blended"—but instead there is space for the client's Self to form a relationship with the part. The answer to this question reveals either enough Self energy to proceed or the presence of another part. If the part cannot step back but instead believes it needs to blend, to take over the client's mind and body, the focus of the session shifts to this new part until it can step aside to allow the client (the client's Self) to form a relationship with the part. Awareness of the client's involuntary movements, voice prosody, and breathing all help the Somatic IFS therapist assess the degree of an embodied, Self-led connection with the part.

> SM: How are you feeling toward this anxious teenager that is showing up in your stomach?
> Tim: Of course I don't like this feeling in my stomach!

His hands leave his stomach and grip tightly on the arms of the chair. It is clear that this response is from a part of Tim. Instead of an explaining, talking manager part we are now hearing from a part that wants to get away from the teenager's feelings. No problem. I bring my Self energy to this part.

SM: This makes sense to me—it must be so uncomfortable. Maybe you and I can help both your stomach and the boy to feel better.

Tim seems to consider this for a couple minutes in silence. His breathing slows and deepens.

SM: How are you feeling now toward the stomach tension?
Tim: [*in a deeper, warmer voice*] I'm feeling more patient with it. I'm feeling sorry for the boy. I feel bad for him. He's really an OK kid. I get that he doesn't want me to be a drunk. He just doesn't want to be criticized and controlled.

His hands move again to his stomach.

5. BEFRIENDING THE PART

Tim has made a leap in the process of differentiating from the part. He has established a Self-led relationship with his teenage protector. We can deepen this all-important relationship with this step of befriending the part. We ask how the part feels toward the client, if the part is even aware of the client's Self being present with him. We bring in some of the Somatic IFS practices to anchor this relationship in a physical reality.

SM: I see your hands are on your stomach where you found the teenager. Does he sense your presence through your hands?

Tim nods yes.

SM: Do you have a sense if your hands are saying something? Either to your gut or to the boy, or maybe both?

Tim breathes deeply into his stomach and moves his hands around.

> Tim: My stomach feels better now . . . I am letting the boy know I'm here.
> SM: It may be hard to know, but can you sense how he feels toward you?
> Tim: Well, he is looking at me. It's like he is glad I am here.
> SM: Good. Let him know he can spend all the time he wants with you, feeling your presence with him in his bedroom.
>
> Tim settles back in his chair. His shoulders and arms open outward slightly. I wonder if this is the first time this part realizes Tim is here with him. I feel glad for this teenage part that no longer feels compelled to use all his energies to resist being controlled. I settle back too. I am enjoying this session.

6. ADDRESSING THE PART'S FEARS

Our protector parts are driven by fears, even if they are reluctant to admit it. When we discover their fears we find out about parts they are protecting or parts threatening their ability to do their jobs. Their fears are rooted in the various systems of the body. Once their fears are identified, understood, and appreciated, the part and Self can negotiate a way to address the fears.

> The teenage part has already told Tim about his fears of being controlled by his dad. As this part is getting to know Tim, he may be beginning to sense that Tim, unlike his dad, is not wanting to control and shame him. I want to test this.
>
> SM: Tim, imagine you could change your drinking behavior. Really envision yourself going through your day in this new way. What happens in your body?
>
> He once more points to his upper abdominal area.
>
> SM: OK, this teenager might still be objecting to this idea.
> Tim: Yeah, he's afraid we'll screw up again.
> SM: Bring your hand to this place you pointed to. Let your breath come to it. Are there any words you want to say to the boy?
> Tim: We have help now. I think it's worth another go of it.

I see his breath come deeper into his stomach, and his jaw and shoulders relax a bit. At least for now, it seems this adolescent part is OK with us getting to know more of Tim's inner system. In later sessions we use these same steps to work with several other protectors. We get to know Tim's part that brought him to therapy, and it comes to trust Tim with the drinking behavior. Then we find, focus, and flesh out the part that uses alcohol and what it fears would happen—in other words, whom it is protecting. These protectors allow us to make contact with the vulnerable parts that hold his pain.

In Somatic IFS we consider the same categories of parts as in IFS—the protectors, which include managers and firefighters, and the more vulnerable ones, called exiles because most often they have been exiled for their own or the system's protection.

Protector Parts and the Body

Protector parts use whatever is at hand to get their jobs done. The body is always there, and protectors use the body and the body's energies. Addictive behaviors, self-harming behaviors, weight loss or gain, acute or chronic illness, muscle tension, dissociation, and pain may be the work of a protector simply trying its best to keep the system from perceived harm. Any healthy or necessary behavior—exercise, eating, sleeping, sex, touch, breathing, even altruistic caring for others—can be enlisted by the part to protect itself, other parts, or the internal system. Like good investors, they can diversify. Like football players, they are strategic. They can block, push, run, tackle, counter, and pass. They are creative. They know how to build effective walls to keep out and to imprison. They can turn the body into a fortress by blocking or buttressing energies at the joints, in the diaphragms, in the lower back. They get hold of our internal pharmaceuticals. They send hormones to affect heart and breath rates. They do what they have to do to keep the individual from getting hurt or being overwhelmed by past hurts. The therapist keeps in mind that any of these physical signs may indicate the behavior of a protector part.

One of the most unique and transformational assumptions of IFS is that all parts have a positive intention. Even though the result of their jobs may be extremely destructive to their own bodies and to others, they all mean well. These protectors came about because of necessity. Often the behaviors they adopted were the best possible response to an impossible situation. They developed as a result of overwhelming pain and they helped the system survive. Weight gain might be an attempt to protect the tender core from repeated boundary violations, or to prevent unwanted sexual interest. Weight loss may be an effort to provide a sense of control. There are parts that hate and fear the body. They may perpetrate, neglect, judge, numb, or immobilize the body. There are parts that use the powerful energies and hungers of the body as their resources for their various functions, and they may deplete, wear out, or kill the body if necessary. Sexual arousal, overeating, and self-mutilation may prevent exiles from overwhelming the other parts.

If the protector part's job is to contain, suppress, hold, and control, it may use the muscles and fascia. They can more easily manage the energies at the demarcation places—any of the joints, pelvic and respiratory diaphragms, throat and jaw, shoulders, and lower back. Other protector parts see their job as action. They activate the endocrine and nervous systems toward "fight or flight" with an increase in heart and breath rates and a release of the stress hormones, or they use another aspect of the autonomic nervous system to dissociate or distract from intense emotion.

Protector parts may use physical symptoms or illnesses to perform their functions. Our burdened parts have admitted that they can make us sick. They seem to be able to deliberately affect our biological systems in order to do their jobs, to tell their stories, or to ask for help. They can use genetic predispositions or organ weaknesses. Parts admit to this, even to being able to obstruct the effects of medications if they believe the disease is important to the person's survival, obviously and paradoxically endangering it. They are too young to understand the consequences. They need our help, not our blame. As we help them, if the physical or mental symptom is from a part, it is improved or healed. One client with chronic fatigue heard from a part that it used this illness to get care and rest for an exiled part. A client with environmental illness has discovered that a part believes it is the only way to protect her from the Cult. The part believes her illness keeps her too sick for them to want her.

Although not all physical conditions can be causally related to parts' roles, when medical interventions are unsuccessful it is important to explore the role of parts in the inner system, as with my client Marco.

Marco has been experiencing chest pains. Although in his early thirties, he is afraid these pains mean he has heart disease. He was referred to me by his doctor, who did not find any related medical cause for his heart pains. A former gang member, Marco is afraid he could easily slip back into the gang culture if he doesn't keep up a tremendous effort. He feels that efforting part as a strong beat in his heart.

With the permission of his parts, I gently place my hand on his chest. His heart is beating so strongly that my entire arm and hand resonate with the beat. I ask him to speak for his heart. In addition to the efforting part, Marco speaks of his tender connection to his mother and of the shame and ridicule he experienced from his older brothers for being a "mama's boy." I respond to his heart's story with compassion, with both words and touch. His heartbeat changes to a normal, gentle lub-dub. He notices it too—he doesn't hear his heartbeat drumming in his ears. I try to guide him to touch his heart and talk to it in a similar way as I hold my hand over his, but his heart, not yet free of his battling protectors, resumes its extreme pattern.

Marco's heart is a battlefield of parts. His managers include the part trying to keep him free of gang culture, his part worrying about his heart health, and a part trying to avoid his brothers' ridicule. His firefighters view his vulnerability as an extreme threat to surviving on the streets of Chicago's west side, so they bind his heart tightly to keep his vulnerable part locked safely away. Marco experiences these warring parts as though he is having a heart attack. In a way, that is exactly what it is—an attack on his heart.

As we bring understanding and compassion to his protector parts, the tender energy in his heart is unburdened from the shame and able to flow freely. His protectors come to learn that he, Marco, is strong, competent, and brave, and all the energy tied up in their efforts is now Marco's as he moves through his life with more Self energy. Not only is he able to resist the pull to return to the gang, but also he goes on to develop a program in high schools for young men of color, which has now expanded to over sixty schools.

As the client and therapist work collaboratively with the protectors, these protectors experience our Embodied Self energy through our relaxed and centered postures, our eye contact, our voice, our breath, and our touch. It is often said that "actions speak louder than words" and "the body does not lie." Along with verbal explanations and reassurances that they are understood and appreciated, our protective parts are using their inherited, adaptive, "Clever Hans" sensitivities to know when they are safe. They are quite clever at determining how to please us and how to resist being hurt in relationships as they have been hurt in the past. They will keep us away from the vulnerable parts, the ones that hold the key to their deepest healing, until the autonomic nervous system has perceived that it is now safe to do so.

Working with Exiles

When the protectors feel understood, exiles often spontaneously show up. Having been banished to an isolated corner of the inner system for their own and the whole system's protection, and now finally sensing an opening, the exiles break through. They are desperate to show and tell of their hurts, their shame, and their unmet needs. The therapist, knowing that releasing these exiles' burdens is the key to unlocking the Self energy in the system, welcomes these parts. The Somatic IFS therapist also knows that working with exiles requires a different approach. While protectors use the body to do their jobs, exiles use the body to tell their stories, either directly or indirectly. When the stories are fully heard, the exiles are restored to their rightful place in the system, allowing the entire system to reorganize. The challenge in working with these vulnerable parts is the intensity of their emotions and sensations. Embodied Self energy provides a safe and compassionate container for them.

With these vulnerable exile parts, even more than with the protectors, the Somatic IFS therapist relies on nonverbal communication. Often their wounds from relational trauma occurred long before they had the capacity to consciously remember, long before they had the words to tell their stories. If these wounds occurred any time from conception through the first four or five years of life, the client's story of the pain or disruption will be told through the body's sensations and movements and disruptions in sensation and movement.

There are additional reasons why the exiles' stories may not be available as a coherent verbal narrative. With later trauma, if the perpetrator has threatened them if they tell of the abuse, their verbal story and even images may be cut off. All that remains of the story are disturbing, intrusive physical symptoms and disruptions in their relationships. Trauma often results in fragmentation of the various aspects of our parts and will inhabit various aspects of the brain, body, and psyche. The painful event may be stored in the reptilian brain, whose language is sensation and movement. The somatic aspect of a part may be cut off from the feelings, thoughts, and images of the event. Sometimes the images and thoughts have been deeply suppressed and only fragments of the body story are available. Many survivors of sexual abuse have cut their body awareness off at the waist, so they aren't overwhelmed by sensations from the abuse. One client only had olfactory memories of her sexual abuse, and these memories intruded on her daily life. Other aspects of that part, the emotional or cognitive or visual, may eventually emerge as the somatic part is compassionately witnessed, yields its burdens, and is restored to its rightful role.

Sometimes, though, the body story of the exiles is dissociated from the rest of the trauma story. While the suppressed body story might only be evident in various debilitating physical symptoms, the trauma may arise in emotional outbursts, disturbing images, or nightmares. The fragmentation of the disparate aspects of the exile's experience means that the therapist works with the most available channel and proceeds with sensitivity and delicacy to integrate the emotions, thoughts, images, and eventually the dissociated body sensations to complete the part's story.

When the emotions of the exiles flood the system, shifting away from the emotions and the verbal narration to focus solely on the body sensations often helps with emotional regulation. Awareness of their feet on the floor, their breath coming in and out calms the emotions. Exiles tend to overwhelm. Emotional regulation is not their strong suit. I sometimes say to my students and clients that exiles have only an on/off switch and we need to help them see that they have a dimmer switch. They need to trust that when we ask them to dial down their intensity we are not trying to trick them back into their dungeons. If the exiles' feelings and behaviors are too intense, the protectors will step in to interrupt the therapy. We ask the exiles to share their story slowly, one piece of the puzzle at a time, so they can re-story the trauma. We reassure them we want to help them safely share the whole story, and we won't forget about them again.

As long as the exile is stuck in the time and in a place where the wounding happened, it may not feel safe to share its story. Instead, the exile will continue to experience an endless repetition of emotions of terror, rage, or shame, and it will continue to perceive the world and people as dangerous, as incapable of giving it the nourishment and support it needs, and of itself as powerless. The exile needs to be retrieved from the past and brought into the present, or into a safe place. Sometimes the exile, recognizing Self energy, will spontaneously leap into the client's lap or more gradually shift into the present. Other times it needs to be more actively retrieved from where it is locked in the basement or hiding in a closet of their childhood home before the system knows the exile is safe to share their story and release their traumatic burdens.

ESTABLISHING A RELATIONSHIP WITH THE EXILE

These vulnerable parts are worked with similarly to protectors in the inner system with a few important differences. The six F steps can be applied to help establish a relationship between the Embodied Self of the client (and/or the therapist) and the vulnerable part. We find, focus, flesh out, and ask the client about their feelings toward the exile. Instead of negotiating with them to step back, we may need to negotiate with the exiles to not overwhelm the system. Exiles tend to take over the system with strong emotions. In IFS we say the part is blended. When exiles blend, they cause the protectors to jump back in, and this can obliterate access to Self energy.

My session with Wendy illustrates bringing Embodied Self energy to her exiled part so she could witness its body story. Wendy had been suffering with painful tension in her jaw and thought it might be related to her sexual abuse. The jaw pain led her to a young girl standing in her playpen, looking out with big, sad eyes. As I asked Wendy how she felt toward this part, one protector after another appeared. Her protectors were not willing to let us connect with this toddler. Her body was held tightly and her breath was very shallow. She was willing to have me guide her with touch and movement to soothe her protectors so her Self energy could be available to relate to this toddler.

> SM: Bring your hands back to your belly and bring a deep breath into your belly, feeling the movement there . . . Now bring one hand a little higher, near your diaphragm . . . Now to your heart, feeling your heartbeat and your lungs . . . As you breathe let your body rock with the rhythm. Just a little movement. Let your front body extend, expand, lift up on the inhale, and return to neutral on the exhale. Do that for several breaths, enjoying the gentle rocking.
>
> Wendy does this very slight movement and seems to visibly relax. Wendy's eyes close.
>
> SM: How is this feeling to you as you do this slight rocking movement?
> Wendy: It feels good.
> SM: Tell me more about the good feeling.
> Wendy: I feel calmer, softer, quieter. I also feel some sadness. My jaw is still tight. It aches.
> SM: Can you go back to seeing the toddler in the playpen?
> Wendy: Yes, I see her. She likes the rocking. Now I am holding her. But she feels much younger. I feel like I am holding a baby in my arms.

WITNESSING THE EXILE'S STORY

We decide to shift our attention to this infant part who has already appeared in her arms, not needing to be retrieved from the past. You will notice I continue to use movement as well as resonance and somatic awareness.

> While Wendy continues to hold the infant as she rocks, I find myself rocking along with her. I am happy that Wendy has connected so well with this baby. I'm feeling content, breathing and rocking

along with her. Then I am drawn to the movement in her head as she rocks back and her head lifts up. Her jaw seems locked into moving along with her head. I remember watching babies nurse, noticing that their heads lift slightly up and down as they suck, separate from their mouth and jaw. I get curious about this and wonder if this is an opportunity to deepen into the infant's story.

SM: I don't remember if I have asked you this, Wendy, but did your mother nurse you?
Wendy: No, I got stuck with a bottle.

Although Wendy got the nutrients she needed, the structures of her mouth didn't get what they needed.

SM: Your jaw is showing you that she was missing something important to her.
Wendy: [*tearing up*] This is what I get and I have to make do.
SM: Let's see if we can help your jaw to experience the movement it missed out on because this baby didn't get to nurse.

Although Wendy's infant part was not frozen in the past in time and location, she was frozen in her physiology, her jaw tension revealing a missing developmental experience, and perhaps Wendy's word "stuck" reveals the jaw pain was pointing to an infant still waiting for this physiological experience. It was stuck in movement, not able to move independently of her head. The various diaphragms of the body are related, and the tension in her soft palate mirrors the tension in her respiratory diaphragm and her pelvic floor. The breathing and rocking movements that relaxed her lower diaphragms opened a path to releasing the tension in the soft palate and jaw.

Early attachment wounds and later traumatic wounds make a potentially indelible physiological imprint. The physiological signs leave a breadcrumb trail to where the parts are captive, leading us to a physiological retrieval. With trauma in general, during a life-threatening, overwhelming event the nervous system emits a biochemical blast to try to help the person escape or get help. When their actions are unsuccessful, the nervous system goes into shutdown. Endorphins are released. Muscles collapse and become still. Blood pressure and heart rate drop. Sensory organs become numb. Memory access and storage are impaired. All the undischarged biochemical residues that were released from the sympathetic activation of the autonomic nervous system are held in the body. Sensory memories flood the system with somatosensory intrusions. Clients' life stories are often peppered with their exiles' futile attempts to escape this physiological loop.

The act of bringing awareness to these physical symptoms begins the process of a physiological retrieval. The Embodied Self of the therapist alone, or along with the client's, can establish a compassionate connection that can help the client's nervous system shift—from a state of dissociative shutdown, through the failed attempt to escape, and eventually to the part's secure connection that repairs the faulty wiring in the limbic system and restores a healthy physiology.

UNBURDENING

Both protectors and exiles have absorbed feelings, sensations, behaviors, and beliefs as a result of their wounds. We call these "burdens." These burdens keep the parts from doing what they would rather do. It is when the burdens of the exiles are released and the exiles are free of their fear, their shame, their isolation, and their feelings of unworthiness that the protectors realize they are also free to let go of their limitations. The unburdening of the exiles occurs in IFS often in a prescribed way, in certain steps. The burden is found somewhere in or around the body. Then, with permission from the parts, the burden is released to the elements of water, air, earth, or fire, or perhaps to the horizon or to the light. The exiles' original qualities are invited to return to the exile.

In Somatic IFS we follow this unburdening process but invite a less prescribed process to releasing the burdens. In addition we attend somatically to spontaneous unburdenings, which may occur during any of the stages of the therapy, and we address them throughout the session. We track shifts in the autonomic nervous system. We notice eye contact, voice prosody, involuntary movements, gestures, and postural changes. We notice the breath rate and depth. Unburdenings can be observed in changes in the client's somatic state, and even in the therapist's body or in the energetic space around this therapeutic dyad. Each of these shifts can be noted, appreciated, celebrated, savored, and anchored with somatic practices.

In the last part of our session I continue to use awareness, movement, and touch to assist the unburdening.

> I direct Wendy to hold the sides of her face. I talk about the muscles of the jaw and the ligaments of the joint between her jaw and her cranium. She opens and closes her jaw. I have her touch the roof of her mouth with her tongue and smack her lips. She lets her tongue rest heavy in her mouth. As she breathes in and her head tilts back, her hands encourage the jaw to remain steady and not go along with her head. On the exhale, the head comes back home to the jaw.
>
> Wendy continues with this movement and feels more movement and softness in her jaw. As she continues to rock and breathe, I notice even more movement in the joint of her jaw. I say a little more about the soft structures of her body—from her mouth through the organs of her digestive system all the way to the anus. I tell her that this softness of this part of her body can help her access her own softness when she tightens up and feels stuck. She feels this issue with her jaw is not complete, but she is glad that she no longer feels stuck and that her whole body has let go of its tension.

With this infant, we could not have identified in verbal terms the specific burdens of the part that did not get to nurse. But it is clear that the burdens are in the disturbed neuromuscular pattern, in the feeling of sadness connected with the movement and the belief that she "had to make do" with less than what she needed. For Wendy unburdening occurred throughout the process as her body became calmer and soft and as she began to recover the lost nursing pattern. As she began to restore a healthy neuromuscular pattern in her jaw, the burdened emotions and beliefs softened.

INVITATION AND RESTORATION OF LOST QUALITIES

This session restored the connection all along the vertical axis from the pelvic floor to the mouth. This vertical alignment begins in utero and is the foundation for moving out into the mystifying and often overwhelming world of relationship in the horizontal plane. The interruption in this line was repaired with each of the practices of Somatic IFS—awareness, breathing, resonance, movement, and touch (her touch in this case). Restoring the movement pattern of nursing laid the foundation for our later working with the neglected toddler part and the older girl who had been molested.

INTEGRATION

I tell Wendy that in order to anchor this new movement pattern in her body it will be important to practice it in the weeks to come. We talk about how she could do this subtle movement of breathing in while her head tilts back and then returns to the jaw on the exhale— while standing in line, waiting in traffic, and any time she thinks about it. I tell her that if she can practice this every day for about three weeks, the neuromuscular patterns will be reinstated. Wendy begins to find it easier to speak up for what she wants in relationship and to bring her power, her innocence, and her playful sense of humor more fully into her world.

Embodied Self

Although this will be covered in more depth in the final chapter, it is important to have a sense of Embodied Self as the five practices of Somatic IFS explored in this book lead us to this state. In IFS we simply refer to "Self" as our essential, core nature, which is similar to what many spiritual traditions recognize as a state of oneness with the Divine that is, without exception, within every person regardless of the severity of their symptoms. Self energy has the power to heal body, mind, and spirit, and a research study has demonstrated it. The results of a randomized control study of rheumatoid arthritis patients showed that an IFS-based intervention reduced symptoms of pain, depression, and anxiety. The physical functioning of the patients improved, as did their self-compassion, all of which were sustained at follow-up.[2] These findings led in 2015 to the IFS model being recognized as an evidence-based practice.

Obviously Self needs to be embodied for its fullest expression of this power. Just as parts inhabit the body, have bodies, and affect the body, so does Self. Self energy is first and foremost experienced in the body. The experience of Self energy is often described in terms of body sensations, such as warm, tingly, expansive, spacious, flowing, openhearted, light, grounded, centered, spacious, calm, and relaxed. The qualities that depict a person in a state of Self energy are often described by words that begin with the letter C: creative, connected, calm, curious, compassionate, courageous, confident, and clear. When each of these qualities is rooted in the body and expressed somatically, it clearly indicates the presence of Embodied Self energy.

Self energy is on a continuum. When we are tired, sick, challenged, or threatened, our parts may dominate, their energies blending or flooding the system. When the parts take center stage, curiosity and compassion may wait in the wings. When the parts step back we find enough Self energy to clean up the mess they made. We move along the continuum from intolerance to tolerance, to acceptance, appreciation, and maybe even gratitude and cherishing. Embodiment is also on a continuum of experience from disembodied to fully embodied. We begin in an embodied state and we lose much of it. Personal, environmental, and social forces can constrain the full embodiment of Self, shifting the state of embodiment moment by moment. The five practices in combination with the IFS model help the parts perceive it is safe for the Self to return to its true embodied nature, beginning with awareness and acceptance, followed by compassion and curiosity. The energy of Embodied Self is amplified as it joins with other Self energies and extends beyond the skin to connect with the wider Field of Self energy in the universe.

Since it is obvious that Self energy is an embodied state, why risk redundancy by including the adjective? To the degree that language influences thought, the emphasis provided by the adjective "embodied" serves to amend our cultural legacy of exiling the somatic realm. Parts and Self are experienced in both body and mind. The terms "body" and "mind" separate the inseparable. The IFS community typically refers to "Self," but Somatic IFS uses the term "Embodied Self" in order to transcend this dualistic paradigm, and I often refer to the "bodymind" to indicate a unified state where both parts and Self are experienced.

How Somatic Practices Support Embodied Self

A *Peanuts* cartoon shows Charlie Brown in a depressed stance. He says, "The worst thing you can do is to straighten up and lift your head high because then you'll start to feel better." The practices of Somatic IFS address the parts-led physical states that keep us from moving out of depression, as well as every clinical issue, and we do start to feel better. Awareness, breath, resonance, movement, and touch move us along the arc of embodiment and also describe the state of full embodiment. Fully embodied, our body pulsates with awareness. Our easy, full breathing reveals the inextricable oneness our bodymind resonates with. Our movements are integrated and fluid, and the language of our touch is responsive, fluent, and healing. Most of the words that describe the practices, like "awareness," "conscious," "mindful," "attuned," even "radical," point to the importance of paying deep attention to the experience, moment by moment, of our bodymind. Most of the time (80 percent, according to some studies) we are not in the present moment but instead we are either lamenting the past or anxiously anticipating and preparing for the future. In IFS terms, we are in the grip of our burdened parts. Being more fully in the present moment describes the state of Self energy.

Somatic Awareness is a quick indicator of my degree of Embodied Self energy and is often the quickest route back to it. I feel expansive, relaxed, and alert when I am in Self energy, and contracted, tense, or cut off when a part is dominant. Sitting with a client, I take a moment of body awareness. I notice tension in my shoulders. As I bring compassion to the tension, my shoulders rest down. I notice my alignment. With my feet on the floor, my sitz bones on the chair, my head aligned with my spine, I'm not fighting with gravity. My spine gets a millimeter longer. I feel more grounded and more connected with my center. Like Charlie Brown predicted, I feel better, and more able to be present with my client. Although my awareness of my body will fluctuate during the session, I will return to it to notice any tension, fidgeting, or collapse that indicates parts showing up. I can more easily take a full breath. I make a slight adjustment to my posture so my breath can come and go more easily.

I bring consciousness to my breath as a clue to what is happening in my nervous system and as a route back to Embodied Self. When our autonomic nervous system is activated, our breath is rapid and shallow; noticing how we are breathing begins to change both our breath and our nervous systems. I intentionally take a longer and slower exhale, which empties my lungs and makes more space for my inhale. Consciousness of my breathing heightens my awareness of my relationship with the space surrounding me and my client. I remember that as I breathe in, I am breathing in energy from the Field of Self to every cell in my body, and I can breathe that energy out to the space around us.

When bringing my client into my awareness, I continue to be aware of my body sensations and my breathing. Being in Self in the face of extreme parts can be the hardest thing we do as therapists. The feelings and behaviors of many parts can be frightening, revolting, and disgusting to our own parts. Parts that cheat, steal, and intentionally hurt—or the passive forms of collapse, stonewalling, or withdrawing—evoke our fearful and condemning parts. Our clients' parts are showing up in their bodies and our body is resonating with them. As mammals, we are hardwired to be physiological empaths. As therapists we are not exempt from the feelings and behaviors of the burdened parts revealed by our clients. If we deny this resonance, we may recruit our protectors to adopt a thin veneer of Self-like control, masking the deeper urge to cut off. A truly "radical" resonance is required. Acknowledging the resonance, our compassion and curiosity stay intact. Our heart can remain open. Staying grounded, my body can be a lightning rod for intense sensations. My breathing energizes and opens my heart, the seat of compassion. My resonant capacity is now in service of my relationship with my client as my posture, gaze, and tone of voice transmit qualities of Embodied Self energy to support my client's process of healing their bodymind system.

The experiences that have led to the client's burdens are waiting to unfold through movement. The movement story of trauma may be frozen in the body's structure by protector parts. Viewing a body symptom, and perhaps many psychological symptoms, as an interrupted body story, we bring awareness, breath, and resonance to the protectors. We mindfully invite a slight movement to the frozen or numb sensations. As the story thaws out, the emotional expression and thwarted movements from the client's experience sequence through the body and are witnessed by the therapist and the client's Self. Disruptions in early motor development are also revealed through the practice of Mindful Movement. Parts may have affected the ability to reach out for safe connection, to explore, to move forward toward a goal, to say yes to life's experiences. Or movements—gestures, gait, unconscious movements—may reveal interferences in the capacity to turn away from, to move away from, to be able to say no, to establish boundaries. Bringing mindful awareness to these inhibited, fixated, or disrupted movements can restore them to greater ease and well-being. Movement can integrate what has been restored. My Embodied Self is expressed in movements in a right-brain-to-right-brain communication with my client, mostly below the level of conscious awareness.

The use of touch in psychotherapy is controversial. Psychotherapists often feel intimidated and ill-equipped to use touch with clients. They and their regulatory agencies also fear the power of touch to deepen intimacy. Grounded in the other practices of Somatic IFS, however, touch can be a powerful addition to the therapist's toolbox of healing approaches. Touch is direct and immediate. It is a direct transmission of all qualities of Embodied Self energy to the parts inhabiting the body and assists with every step of IFS. Although even with my bodywork background I have some cautious parts regarding touch, I appreciate this modality especially for the wordless stories I hear with my hands, the stories that may not yet be able to be told in words or even feelings or images. Attuned Touch is the ultimate right-brain, body-to-body communication. It has the capacity to heal the effects of harmful touch and the lack of necessary touch.

As I write this section of Embodied Self, I stop and notice where I am on the continuum of Embodied Self. Hmmm. More at the lower end. Can I use Somatic IFS to shift this? With a long, slow exhale I turn my attention inward to scan my body for sensations. Of all the sensations I notice—slight tensions in my face and arms from writing—I am drawn to a slight pain in my upper left sacral joint. At first I am distracted by sounds in the room, but as I refocus I feel a wave of energy up my spine and down my arms. My spine wants to move now. As I move, I notice a place in the mid-back on the right that feels stuck. As I explore the depth and the boundaries of that stuck place, another rush of energy follows. My whole torso feels more spacious and my sense of the shape of my torso expands and the boundaries get blurry. The whoosh of energy travels up the back of my neck. My shoulder blades drop a bit further down my back. My breath gets longer and slower and my spine begins to move with my breath. I notice tension behind my eyes and at the base of my throat. As I stay with that tension, I feel a wave of energy, like an internal shower, flowing down my back into my pelvis and down the back of my legs. I continue to ride the wave of my breath. I feel more alive, more spacious. I say "I" but this experience of sensation and movement shifting moment by moment is the reality rather than a concept of "I."

Introduction to the Following Chapters on the Five Practices of Somatic IFS

In the chapters to follow, each of these practices will be explored and integrated with IFS to investigate the internal system through the physiology and the felt sense of the body. We will look at how experiences shape the brain and the body and how symptoms, body structure, and body processes reveal parts. We will learn how our social brain heals attachment wounds. I will describe experiences that have led me to understand that a more fully embodied Self is a resource for leading the system toward a life that is more fully lived. We include the conceptual aspects of the somatic work—the why and the how.

Just as the goal of IFS is to free up the Self of the individual to lead their internal system, the goal of Somatic IFS is to restore an Embodied Self. The foundational tool is **Somatic Awareness.** The logo for Somatic IFS illustrates that this practice embraces all the rest, supporting them, almost as if this practice is giving birth to the other practices. Practically speaking, awareness of the body naturally leads to awareness of the breath, so the next practice is **Conscious Breathing.** On top of that is **Radical Resonance,** where we move more fully into the relational realm. **Mindful Movement** can be explored within the context of the relational field, and **Attuned Touch** is at the apex, occupying the least amount of space, yet in some ways it is the most powerful. Each practice is interdependent. Each one alone can possibly lead to the state of Embodied Self, but the sequence and interaction of the five practices multiplies the potency of each practice.

Even though these five practices are considered separately, it will become obvious that the lines are blurred and are, in some cases, nonexistent. Somatic Awareness is not a practice that is used and then abandoned as we move into the other practices; rather it is the basis of all the other practices. The same can be said for all the other seemingly separate practices. Along with the separate steps of the IFS model, and the categorization of our internal worlds into manager, firefighter, exiles, and Self, the five practices of Somatic IFS provide a useful map in navigating the mysterious territory of the bodymind.

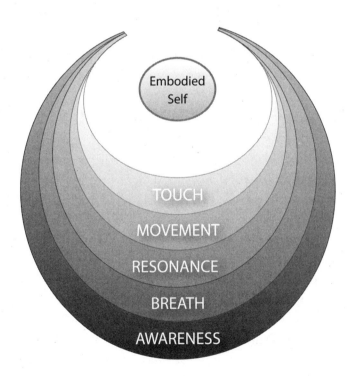

Each practice is associated with an element from classical Greek thought: earth, air, fire, and water. The IFS therapist is already familiar with using these classical elements with the step of unburdening. In this step of the IFS process, the therapist will ask the client's parts which of the elements it wants to use to let go of the burden. While unburdening in Somatic IFS is less prescribed, these basic elements are one way to understand the nature and complexity of the body and of all our material world. The classical elements provide us with one lens from which to consider our body and our relationships with the external world, which is essential in therapy. They also offer an opportunity to experience the practice at its most fundamental level.

Particular body systems are also explored in each chapter on a Somatic IFS practice. The body systems are an additional way to understand the body's complexity as well as to appreciate the systemic nature of the bodymind. All the body systems, like all the practices, are interdependent. Although understanding a body system in depth may not be immediately clinically applicable, I have found my study of anatomy and physiology and even embryology to be a relevant and crucial underpinning for my bodymind therapeutic interventions, as will become clear in my case examples.

Classical Elements Associated with the Five Practices

In classical thought, the four elements—earth, air, water, and fire—are considered to be the basis of all matter and the archetypal forces of creation. These elements have provided the foundation of medicine, philosophy, and science for millennia, constituting the basis of many ancient healing practices. The therapeutic approaches of many cultures have considered the relationship of these elements to physical, emotional, and spiritual symptoms to alleviate and cure an array of human ailments. Their accumulated healing wisdom that has contributed to our survival as a species still informs many of our effective therapeutic and restorative approaches. Although modern science has vastly expanded our therapeutic repertoire, these elemental forces and sensory experiences link our current modalities to healing legacies from our ancestors.

Hippocrates associated the four elements with the four humours. Carl Jung derived his theory of personality types from these four humours, associating personality types with them. The four elements of earth, air, fire, and water became the cornerstone of medieval alchemical healing practices. In Buddhism these elements are viewed as categories of sensory experience and are considered a basis for understanding suffering and for liberating ourselves from suffering.

The IFS therapist employs the four elements to facilitate the most transformative aspect of therapy—the step that liberates our parts from their suffering—the unburdening process. The client, or the client's part, when it is ready to let go of its burden of emotion, perception, or belief, is asked which of the four elements it would like to release the burden to. Some reply they will bury it deep in the earth where it can be composted. Others will release it to the air where it can dissipate into the infinite space above and around us. Some burdens are consumed by fire where they are reduced to ashes, while others sail away in the ocean or are cleansed in a waterfall. Released in this way to the elements, the quintessential, incorruptible, spiritual aspect of the individual is freed to emerge in the internal system. Balance and harmony among the parts is established by this transcendent spiritual essence we call "Self," this experience of a state of being that indeed is a quantum leap from the experience of burdened parts with their fear-driven strategies for survival. The archetypal aspects of the four elements are infused in our experience of Embodied Self energy.

These four elements have an even larger place in Somatic IFS. These basic elements connect us with the larger universe—the ground below our feet, the air surrounding us, the life-giving waters, the fire that warms our heart and lights our way. As we listen to heart-wrenching tales from our clients, we feel our feet, gaze out the window at the sky, drink our tea, glance at a candle. Each element deepens our experience with its associated Somatic IFS practice.

I associate Somatic Awareness, as the foundation of all the other practices, with the element earth. We bring our awareness to the floor or the chair below us and connect with the earth, allowing our energies to ground and center. We appreciate how the earth has abundantly supported us, how we have planted seeds and harvested during our lifetimes. We walk in the footsteps of so many who have walked the earth before us. We are grounded and supported every step of the way. The earth knows the rhythms and cycles of change, the mountainous heights and the deep darkness of caves. Connecting again and again to the earth we develop a dependable anchor in the face of tumultuous emotional energies. Perhaps we can assist our clients to find safety and support from the earth, to trust that even their deepest secrets and darkest fears can become fertile soil for tender new seeds to flourish. Anchored to our home base we look to the infinite sky above.

Conscious Breathing connects us with the air element as we bring our awareness to this largely unconscious act. The air element connects us to earth and to sky through our vertical alignment and reveals that at the most basic level we are mostly empty space. Spaciousness is one of the main descriptors of Self energy. When in the grip of parts our energies tighten and narrow, become denser, more constricted. The rhythms of respiratory and cellular breathing create calm and spaciousness within our body and mind. Each inbreath brings new possibilities, new life. Each outbreath allows us to let go of what we no longer need, making space for the new. Breathing is the bridge between inner and outer worlds. Awareness of the exchange of our inner and outer systems unites us with the entire world of aerobic life.

Our breath leads us to the relational realm of Radical Resonance. Associated with the element of water, this practice involves resonating through our heart and our fluid systems with the experiences of others. The element water is associated with emotions, fluid movement, and transformation. Water is soothing, nourishing, cleansing, and purifying. Our parts thirst for resonant, compassionate witnessing of the injustices that corrupted our innocence and dried up our dreams. The healing rivers of compassion stream from our heart and mind to water the parched soil of our inner landscapes. We find the courage to dive into the deep end of the pool. A resonant relationship assists in navigating emotional waters as we reverberate through our heart and our largely fluid body.

Mindful Movement connects us with the element fire. Fire is associated with energy, growth, and transformation. With mindful attention, the warmth of movement thaws the frozen tundra of trauma; what begins as a sensation is transformed by the energy of movement to a body story of the internal system. The body story might be frozen in tense or collapsed tissues, awaiting the warming thaw of Embodied Self energy to ignite the telling of the body story through voluntary and involuntary movement. The movement might be a small gentle flame or a large expressive story of the body.

Attuned Touch incorporates these elements, involving the interplay of earth, air, water, and fire. All the qualities of the elements come together for touch to be a safe, reciprocal communication. The vertically aligned therapist connects with the heart. The compassionate warmth of the physical contact resonates with the tissues and communicates Self presence. Wounds from abuses and neglect of touch can be healed by Attuned Touch. Physically communicating Embodied Self energy relies on all the elements and all the practices to ensure it will be a tool for profound healing.

Just as Ayurvedic medicine and traditional Chinese medicine consider the interrelationships among the elements to diagnose and treat imbalances in the body, mind, and spirit, the elements associated with Somatic IFS and the five practices of Somatic IFS are dynamic and interrelational. We sit with our client and connect with the earth and make shifts in our posture so we are not fighting with gravity. The energies from the earth are more available to flow through us. We notice we are breathing. We allow our bellies to soften and our breath to deepen. Feeling solid and grounded as well as spacious and open, we can now enter the horizontal plane of where we can "go with the flow" of relational interactions. If we get swept away in the rising rapids of emotion, connecting with the fluids of our body might help us skillfully flow around the rocks in the stream. If our receptive systems are flooded, we come back to ourselves—our connection to heaven and earth—through awareness of sensation and breath. The fire of movement brings warmth, light, and energy to the therapy process. Movement depends on awareness, breath, and resonance to support its most authentic expression. A client's breath, movement, or touch might be a starting point for exploring the internal system, and at times in a session there may be a confluence of all the practices in an interaction. The four elements remind us of our need for balance and our interdependence. When in balance we are connected with the infinite Field of Self energy.

Body Systems Associated with the Five Practices

Along with each of the four elements, certain body systems are associated with each of the five practices of Somatic IFS. Of course, every part of the body is relevant when working with the bodymind—every body system, every organ, joint, muscle, and bodily process. IFS is based on systems theory that recognizes the interrelationships and interdependence of the parts and the Self with the external environment. The body is also understood as a cohesive collection of body systems made up of cells, tissues, and organs, organized along their functions, such as the respiratory, digestive/excretory, nervous, musculoskeletal, endocrine, and cardiovascular systems. These systems, both in IFS and in the body, have predictable behaviors, are dynamic, and have constraints. Each system has a job to do and communicates with other systems. Changing one part of the system affects other parts, or the whole system. Each system has qualities of Self energy, like intelligence, creativity, and resilience. Parts will use these body systems to do their jobs and to communicate their stories.

Linda Hartley talks about experiencing these anatomical systems through the practices of Body-Mind Centering as she references Roberto Assagioli's psychosynthesis methods. "They might be felt to embody inner 'characters,' the subpersonalities or constellations of energy that coexist within us, acting and interacting with each other in patterns unique to every individual. These patterns may at times remain fixed, or they may change and reorganize themselves into new relationships as our life unfolds."[3] Susan Aposhyan of Body-Mind Psychotherapy has written extensively about many body systems from a psychological point of view.[4] Touching into these body systems contacts parts and invites them to unfold. Their emotions, beliefs, and histories are witnessed through awareness and movement. As they are fully witnessed the systems can reorganize toward greater wellness and harmony.

Although every system of the body can be considered with each of the five practices of Somatic IFS, some have a strong association to each practice. For the basic practice of Somatic Awareness we consider the skeletal, fascial, and nervous systems. Bones are the densest of the body's tissues. We connect with the earth through our pelvic sitz bones and our feet. The fascia forms our total structure, uniting us from head to toe, from inside to outside. The nervous system transmits and makes sense of the sensory information. We bring awareness to these parts of our body to ground us, to stabilize us, to connect us to the ground of our being.

Conscious Breathing involves our lungs, circulatory system, and muscles of respiration. A more subtle respiration is occurring within each cell through its membrane. Both pulmonary and cellular respiration involve an interchange, a connection between inside and outside. Both kinds of respiration provide rhythmic cycles that bring calmness and clarity.

The practice of Radical Resonance involves our central nervous system, including our autonomic nervous system and the structures of our limbic brain. It also considers the heart as not just a simple mechanical pump for our blood but also an emitter of an electromagnetic field far more powerful than that of the brain. A compassionate, open heart and mind in relationship have the power to revise the hearts and minds of others. Radical Resonance engages the fluid systems of the body—the blood, the lymph, the extracellular matrix surrounding all of our cells passing through the cell membrane, and the fluid within our joints and bathing our brain and spinal cord. Tuning in to our bodily fluids we find the wisdom of containment, boundaries, and the reciprocal flow of connection.

Mindful Movement involves the physical sources of our movement impulses from the subtle to the gross, including our muscular system, our somatic nervous system, and our autonomic nervous system. Our voluntary and unconscious movements arise out of the intentions and desires fueled by the emotions stored in any of our tissues. Our muscular system embodies qualities of creativity, courage, and confidence. The practice of Mindful Movement includes the embryological development of the body in utero as a template and as a source of unburdening those faulty movement patterns. The body in relative stillness is moving—contracting and expanding rhythmically with the flow of breath, cerebral spinal fluid, blood, and digestive processes.

Attuned Touch engages the skin and the sensory nerves, which together make up the somatosensory system. From the surface of our skin, information is sent through various sensory receptors and neurons to the spinal reflexes, then to the unconscious brain stem, and finally to the fields of awareness of the cortex. This system is a two-way street, with information flowing in both directions simultaneously. The body tissues perceive, receive, and respond to the qualities of Embodied Self energy implicitly communicated through the hands of the client, the therapist, or both.

Each system of the body reflects multiplicity. From the simplest molecule to the entire body, each aspect reveals a constantly evolving functioning intelligence, vast creativity, and amazingly effective communication and collaboration. The body strives for homeostasis among its various parts. Forces—internal and external—can disrupt that balance. Parts' polarizations and oppositional stances may be reflected in imbalances in the musculoskeletal structure, in dysregulated nervous systems, or in suppressed or unbalanced endocrine function.

The path to Embodied Self energy—the goal of Somatic IFS—is accomplished through exercising these five practices and their associated elements and body systems. At the end of every chapter are exercises for experiencing the topics covered in the chapter. Each exercise is followed by suggestions for reflecting on your experience. Most of the exercises are intended to be done individually and a couple of them require a partner. The intention of these exercises is to provide a safe experience of embodying the somatic practice and to deepen your connection with the parts in your internal system through that particular practice. As you do the exercises you will want to attend to the level of activation of your parts. If your protective parts cause you to feel distracted, bored, or critical, or if your vulnerable parts begin to flood your system with their emotions or beliefs, you can come back to an earlier exercise that helped you access your Embodied Self energy. Once you are familiar with the exercises that have facilitated your awareness of your own embodied internal family, integrating these practices in your clinical work will help your clients and patients deepen their own Embodied Self energy.

EXERCISES

Parts in the Body

PURPOSE   To find parts in the body; to identify if they have burdens and, if so, what the burdens are. To identify them as either protector parts or vulnerable parts.

INSTRUCTIONS:

1. Lying or sitting, bring your awareness to an experience in your body.

2. Focus on this place in your body. Stay with the sensation(s).

3. As you stay with the sensation, consider if there are words that go with it. If it could speak to you, what would it say? What does it want?

4. Is there an emotion that seems to be at the heart of this sensation or that seems to connect with the words? What is the feeling(s)?

5. If these experiences of sensation, words, and emotion lead to a part, perhaps the part also wants you to see it, to know its age, its gender, where it is.

6. Ask yourself if you feel open and curious toward this part. If so, let the part know this is how you feel—in words, in your body energy, in your touch. If not, find this part in your body and start again with step 2.

7. If the part responds and is willing to talk with you, let it know you are listening.

8. As you hear from the part, you may have a sense of the category of the part. If the part is using your body for its job, it is a protector. If it is using the body to tell you its story, it is a vulnerable part.

9. Thank the part for being willing to share with you.

REFLECTIONS   (journal, draw, or share with a partner)

1. What was the sensation?

2. Where was it in your body?

3. Did it lead to a part? If so, how did you feel toward the part?

4. What did you learn about the part?

5. Could you tell if the part was a protector or a vulnerable part?

6. Do you have a sense what the part needs from you?

WORKING WITH PROTECTOR PARTS THROUGH THE SIX FS

When we are in a state of Embodied Self energy, the words to say to the client emerge easily. But when we're first learning, suggested scripts can be useful in helping the client move through the six Fs of Somatic IFS therapy.

1. Finding a Part

These suggested statements and questions are intended to help the client turn their attention toward the information being communicated from their inner system. The therapist listens to the client's verbal and nonverbal language and responds:

- To a thought: "So, it sounds like a part of you is (thinking/ believing) ___?"

- To a physical sensation: "Could this _____ sensation in your body be a part wanting your attention?"

- To a posture, gesture, movement: "I am noticing ___. I wonder if this is the way a part is communicating with us right now."

- To an emotion: "I hear (or see) that a part of you is feeling __."

- To memories/images: "Is this image coming from a part of you?" "Is a part of you showing you this memory?"

2. Fleshing Out a Part

The intention of this step is to help the client know the part as fully as possible, as a subpersonality with a body, feelings, beliefs, and behaviors. Depending on the client's response, the therapist relies on their own somatic experience and the client's nonverbal communication to ask questions or make observations that help the client attain a more thorough experience of the part. The general idea is to help the client begin to get to know their part more fully. Protectors often use the body—the body's systems, energies, behaviors—to do their jobs, so it is important to include the sensations and movement impulses of the part.

- With parts that first appear as thoughts:
  - "As you listen to this thought, notice if there are any feelings that go along with it."
  - "Say your thought aloud and notice if there is any change in your body."
  - "As you hear this part say these words, what happens to the wall around your heart?"
  - "As I hear your words, I am aware of _____ happening in your body."
- With parts that first appear as physical sensations and movements:
  - "As you stay with this agitation, notice if there are any thoughts (words/emotions/images/memories) that go along with it."
  - "If this numbness in your body could speak, what would it say?"
  - "Does the tension in your jaw want to move or speak?"
- With parts that first appear as an emotion:
  - "Where in your body is this fear?"
  - "Does this angry part want to move?"
  - "Does this feeling have any words/memories/images?"
- With parts that first appear as memories/images:
  - "Stay with this image and notice what is happening in your body."
  - "As you look at this image, are you aware of any feelings?"

3. Focusing on a Part

This step may precede "fleshing out." The statements are directions but could be restated as a question, such as "Would you be willing to . . . ?" The intention of the statement or question is to support the continuation of the client's open, curious attention on their part. In particular, staying focused on the physical sensations often helps the client unblend from intense emotions and from narrating and analytical protector parts.

- "I'd like to hear more about that, but for now can you just stay with the heavy stone in your heart?"
- "Keep looking at this image of the warrior. Can you see his face? What is he wearing?"
- "Is the tension in your stomach mostly on the surface, or does it go all the way through to your back? Are the edges of it clear or blurry? Is there movement in the tension or is it static?"
- "Keep moving in this way and notice what happens."

4. Asking How the Client Feels toward the Part

This step helps to differentiate the part and Self. This step also may come earlier in the process.

- Answers from the client that reveal a part:
  - "I don't like it. I wish it would go away."
  - "I feel sorry for it." (This one may indicate a pitying part, but it could also indicate compassion.)
  - "I think it will never stop doing ____."
  - "The part has been around a long time."
  - Nonverbal language (involuntary movements, posture, voice prosody, breathing, facial expression), despite the verbal answer, may reveal the presence of a part instead of Self energy.
- The therapist asks the part if it can step back. If not, this part becomes the new "target" protector part until it can step back.

- Answers that reveal Self energy:
  - "I would like to get to know it better."
  - "I would like to help it trust me."
  - "I'm glad to hear from this part."
  - "I feel warm toward him."
  - "I'm open to hearing more from her."
  - "I'm wondering what he needs from me to be able to rest."

5. Befriending the Part

- For the Self-to-part relationship the therapist asks:
  - "Where do you feel this compassion in your body?"
  - "Where in your body do you feel this warmth?"
  - "What in your body lets you know you feel curious?"
- The therapist directs the client to send this sensation of Self energy to the part.
- For the part-to-Self relationship the therapist asks:
  - "Is the part aware of you?"
  - "Does the part seem willing to sense into whether or not you are trustworthy?"
  - "What happens to him when you surround him with warmth from your heart?"
  - "Does she seem interested in letting you get to know her better?"
  - "Is the part looking at you now that you have said those words to him?"

6. Addressing the Part's Fears

Our protector parts are driven by fears, even if they are reluctant to admit it. They fear what would happen if they did not do their job, and they fear other parts will keep them from doing their jobs.

- The therapist asks the part, or directs the client to ask their part: "What are you afraid would happen if you were not doing ___?"

- The part's response points toward either the vulnerable one it is protecting or another protector that is polarized with it.

- "Where in your body is that fear?"

- Hearing of the fear or concern of the part, the therapist and/or the client responds empathically and appreciatively to the part:

  - "I get that. I agree, that would not be good if that happened."

  - "You have been working hard for a long time at your job, never giving up."

  - "What happens to that place in your body when you hear me say that?"

- Negotiating with the protector part:

  - "If we could help take care of that part/help that interfering part to stop, would you like that?"

  - "Is there something you would rather do (or be) if we could take care of that?"

  - "Can you imagine what that would feel like if you could be that way?"

  - "Is there something you need from me/us to allow you to trust us?"

  - "You can watch from the sidelines and step in if you need to."

2

Somatic Awareness: Reading the Body Story

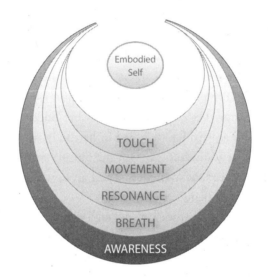

I HOLD MY NEWBORN granddaughter in my arms as she roots around searching for a milk-laden breast. Her eyes are closed, her nose is bobbing, searching left and right, up and down. Not finding a source of lunch on my body, she yawns, sneezes, and sighs. Her fist finds her mouth and she sucks with vigor. Her eyes open and seem to be focusing inward. I nestle her in her familiar fetal position and she relaxes into my arms. I gaze at her closing eyelids and feel her weight and warmth against my body.

I wonder how she is experiencing her new world through her nose, her skin, her ears and eyes. What is her "somatic" experience—her subjective bodily sensations as she transitions from swimming in her warm watery world to moving her spine and her limbs on land? How does she exercise her birthright of somatic awareness, to learn, to grow, to get her needs met? Within minutes of her birth she was weighed, measured. Her vital functions are assessed by a medical team. Unlike this *objective* approach to the body that observes and measures, the term "somatic" refers to one's *subjective* bodily experience.

Over a year later my granddaughter has accumulated a vast amount of bodily experiences that have helped her learn to navigate as a two-legged animal. She totters on the cool, hard, wooden floor. She pauses and then steps onto the soft, dense, wool rug, and pauses again, processing all the information her senses are receiving. I reflect on her efforts to sense and make sense of her world. I muse about what may lie ahead for her as an embodied being on this planet. Will there be support for her fullest embodiment? Will she know herself to be awake to her bodily pleasures, aware of its hungers, and able to feel at home in her body wherever she travels on the planet? Or will interactions with the outside world cause her parts to blunt her innate somatic awareness? I feel an upwelling in my heart to protect this vulnerable being.

Compared to hers, my senses have dulled. I wonder when I last attended so fully to the sensations on the bottom of my feet. Instead I focus on where I am going and how long it will take me to get there and only consider my feet if my shoes are hurting me. Manager parts view my body as an object to get me where I need to go. I make a commitment to ask my parts to allow me to be more present to my moment-by-moment body sensations.

I think of clients whose painful life experiences have blunted their connection to their subjective body experience. They have been neglected, abandoned, and abused. Focusing on their body sensations, sometimes even for a brief moment, elicits overwhelming pain. Clients who have been treated as objects to be used or misused have had their birthright to know their bodies from the inside out ripped from them. Because developing our capacity for awareness is so predictive not only of Self energy but also of our health and happiness, Daniel Siegel has written an entire book about this practice, appropriately titled *Aware*.[1] He cites research that indicates that strengthening our capacity for awareness improves the health of our mind, body, and relationships, including improving immunity and cardiovascular functions and enhancing epigenetic regulation of genes.

Committed to helping my clients restore their bodily awareness, I realize this will require sensitivity and appropriate timing, patience, and persistence. My own capacity for somatic awareness will be crucial in the process of winning the trust of the protective parts that have blocked the body story so that the story can safely unfold and be held with reverence and respect. This practice of Somatic Awareness provides an essential base for a more fully embodied Self energy.

Awareness is central in any healing process. Somatic Awareness involves a focused, open attention to one's bodily experience as it unfolds moment by moment. We notice sensations and lack of sensation. As we separate from parts that reject or criticize the sensation and maintain our awareness, the body story is revealed. As the story is witnessed and the burdens are released, awareness *of* our body increases the awareness *in* our body. We inhabit our body. We are *being* a body rather than *having* a body. Somatic Awareness leads to restoring and cultivating Embodied Self energy.

Looking at the image of the five practices of Somatic IFS, we find Somatic Awareness at the base, laying the framework for the practices to follow. A Somatic IFS therapy session uses each of these practices with every step of the model toward the goal of a fuller access to Embodied Self. The other practices of breathing, resonance, movement, and touch are supported by and embraced by this practice of body awareness. Each of the five practices of Somatic IFS emerge from and depend upon each other. They are sequential and all flow organically from awareness and yet they function interdependently. The course of each session touches back repeatedly on this foundational practice of body awareness.

Somatic Awareness starts the process of healing. Bringing awareness to the sensations in our body we become conscious of our breath. The exchange of air in and out of our body connects our internal sensations with our external environment. This connection ushers in the relational realm where body awareness and our common breath refines our resonant capacity. The parts that use the body sensations to do their jobs or to share their histories are witnessed through a sustained, compassionate awareness. The sensations sequence through the body as their body story is told in movement. The parts' burdens from an objectifying world are found and released from where they were frozen in the depths of the body. The freedom in the body is evident in the restoration of vibrancy, grace, connection, and power.

Obviously if we are only listening to the verbal account, we are missing most of the story. Our clients may have a coherent verbal narrative of their personal histories that they explicitly remember, but what of their histories before they had language? What of the events of their lives that have been exiled, suppressed, and erased from their conscious memories? These stories are waiting to be told through sensations and movement impulses. The thwarted experiences, overwhelming traumas, or faulty attachments that bring our client to seek therapy are revealed before that client even opens their mouth to speak.

Communications experts inform us that 70–80 percent of communication is nonverbal, conveyed through tone of voice, facial expressions, gestures, and posture. If these percentages apply to ordinary human communication, how much more are the depths of our psyche, the implicit memories, and preverbal attachment trauma communicated through the body? For many clients, awareness of the body is the only available channel for their parts and their stories to be known. For other parts, words may accompany the body story, like subtitles in a foreign film. The body, sculpted by history, provides the third dimension to the oral account. If the physical aspect of the part is not evident, if instead the part first shows itself to us as a thought, image, or emotion, we invite the part to be known in its fleshed-out fullness. To miss the body story of the part is to be missing most of the show.

As I am writing this, I get a call from a client standing outside my office door who thought we had a session. I thought I had communicated that I would not be in town, but most likely I am at fault and there's nothing I can do about it. I picture her waiting outside my door for me to open it and greet her, and I hear the disappointment and annoyance in her voice.

I feel a sensation in my upper chest, like a heavy weight pressing inward. I ignore it and continue with my writing, but the weight is hard to ignore.

Again I try to get away from the heaviness and come up with words to label the emotions. Finally, I just stay with the heaviness. I ask the distracting parts to let me just be with the sensations. They are OK with me turning from my computer and listening to my body. The heaviness pulls my head down, and the heaviness in my upper chest travels down my core toward my belly. There is a sense of something wanting to flower. I feel a prickly sensation behind my eyes, like the beginning of tears. Again I notice a distracting part, telling me this is enough, that I have a book to write. I let the part know that it is important for me to be with this feeling as long as it needs my attention.

The sensation—heavy, dark, dense—begins to lighten, and I hear this part urging me to find a way to repair the rupture. This relationship matters a great deal to me. I have a thought to offer my next session for free. With that idea, sensations that I describe as an internal shower flow down my arms and along the sides of my face. My inbreath allows my chest and head to rise. I turn back to my computer and send her a text, and the inner shower flows again. When she accepts my gesture, it feels like all my cells are sparkling in waves up and down my body.

Awareness *of* the Body and Awareness *in* the Body

A simple experiential exercise I share at the beginning of a Somatic IFS workshop reveals the inherent awareness waiting to be uncovered. I ask participants to notice one of their hands. After a few minutes of attending to the sensations of the skin, muscles, bones of our hand we then compare that hand with the other one. Participants describe the hand they were aware of as warmer, larger, more tingly, more relaxed, more sensitive and alert. They had inhabited their hand from the inside rather than observing it from the outside. It's a simple way to demonstrate that awareness *of* leads to awareness *in* our body. The participants want the other hand, and even their whole body, to feel this way. Awareness alone is transformative. Combining it with IFS is life-changing.

Cultivating our capacity for awareness of our body is a lifetime endeavor. As therapists we begin, of course, with awareness of our own sensory experience in order to detect parts so we can return to the state of Embodied Self energy. We turn our attention to our body sensations. As we notice our sensations, typically parts immediately arise—parts that assess, judge, or want to change our experience. If instead we can be aware *of* these bodily sensations, and we can center our attention *within* the sensations, the awareness itself is transformative. Awareness *within* the sensation reveals the intrinsic awareness in every cell and system of our body. This practice helps us fully inhabit our body, to be in our body, to *be* our body.

Sitting with our client, we listen to their compelling verbal story, and we also see that there is another story—the body story—unfolding moment by moment. Without the intention to pay attention we could miss it. While we are listening as intently to the nonverbal stories as the verbal ones, the body story may be told in movement or lack of movement, in posture and stance, in myriad facial expressions, and in subtle shifts in breathing, skin color, and pupil size. The wealth of information is received with curiosity and compassion. The body might tell one story while the mouth contradicts it. Reading the body story is like watching a foreign film. The body story is the actions of the actors and the soundtrack; the verbal story is the subtitles.

It is crucial that it is our Self observing the client's body story. If it is a part doing the observing, we may be analyzing, comparing, criticizing, or interpreting what we are seeing. A distancing manager may be viewing our clients' bodies through a lens of needing to contain or fix. Aware of tensions, holdings, physical discomfort, and areas of our body outside of our awareness, we find our parts, focus on them, and eventually free up our Self energy to be the observer.

As Somatic IFS therapists, if we are not analyzing or interpreting what we are observing, what do we do with all this information? The answer, of course, depends. Sometimes I simply note it and store it, integrating this data with the verbal information. If I sense my client's process will be helped, I may say, "I notice while you are talking, your right shoulder keeps lifting up. Is that something you are curious about?" or "Your body seems to collapse a little when you say that. Can you sense that?" I might suggest more generally turning their attention to what is going on in their body at any point in the session. "What is your body telling you as you try to decide where to go next?" "How is your part using your body to let us know how it feels?"

Inviting the sensations, welcoming them, and deepening the sensory experience facilitates the six Fs of the IFS process. We ask the question that helps determine whether or not there is observing Self energy, "How do you feel toward this sensation?" The questions we ask don't serve our curiosity but are geared to help the client stay focused on and deepen their experience. I may inquire about the kind of sensation, the shape, size, depth. I may ask if there is a direction of the pull of the tension or holding. The answers are less important than whether or not they help the client stay engaged with the sensation. Meanings emerge naturally from the body story and are integrated into the sensate experience. The meanings lead to a fuller understanding of the part's experience as well as information about the beliefs, behaviors, and emotions that are organizing the part's role in the system.

My client may find the sensation too intense. If this happens, protectors will interrupt the body awareness, distracting from or deadening the sensations. These parts don't want us to feel bad. They fear we will never climb out of the pit of bad feeling. They may be trying to balance out parts that amp up the intensity of the pain to make sure they are heard, flooding the system, obliterating the capacity of the Self to be present. The polarization may escalate as the part with the body story becomes more desperate and turns up the volume even more. This tragic irony tends to repeat, as the neural firings become neural connections. The client is trapped in extreme sensorial oscillations. We ask the protector to trust us as we see if the sensation can move into a tolerable range. We can ask the sensation to lessen. We let the part with the body story know we will be able to listen even better if the signal is lower. If it cannot lower the volume, we ask the part to let us know what it would need to be able to do that.

When the sensations are not overpowering, it is often important to the part that we give permission for the full flow of sensation. The process of witnessing the body story is a sequence that begins with noticing, accepting, observing, focusing, deepening, allowing, and finally *being* the sensation, allowing it to fill our awareness. Our parts that are communicating through sensation are no longer isolated. They feel witnessed, respected; and much of the pain they hold from being alone, ignored, and vilified by other parts in the system is resolved. The flow of Embodied Self energy is restored.

The situation I described where I stood up my client illustrates this sequence. My blocking protectors relaxed back and I noticed, accepted, and observed the sensations. I kept my focus on the sensation of heaviness and it deepened and expanded. I beheld the heaviness in all its weight and darkness. The underlying sadness was revealed along with a Self-led response that brought very pleasant sensations to my body and resulted in a repair and a deepening of the relationship with my client.

Awareness Involves Different Kinds of Perception

Different kinds of awareness are described by words that have the suffix "-ception": interoception, exteroception, and proprioception. The practice of Somatic Awareness involves all of them—developing and making more conscious these different ways of knowing our bodymind. Somatic Awareness also considers that these sensory capacities can be disturbed and distorted by trauma and can be restored through Somatic IFS.

"Interoception" refers to the awareness of our subjective physical experience—the therapist and client tuning in to their inner body sensations to identify their feeling states. We use our interoceptive awareness to attune to the various sensations and movement impulses in our body. Sensory nerve endings receive signals from our gut, heart, and other internal organs and body tissues that influence the feelings, moods, and thoughts of our parts and are the basis of our subjective sense of ourselves. Many affective neuroscientists have related interoceptive awareness with emotional and cognitive processes and see interoception as a key element in our understanding of the bodymind. Disruptions in interoceptive awareness and interoceptive sensitivity show up in emotional and physical illnesses. Heightened interoception shows up in panic and anxiety disorders, while suppressed interoception shows up in post-traumatic stress disorder (PTSD) and depression.

Developing our interoceptive capacity gives us more access to our Self energy. A study of fibromyalgia patients and interoception suggests that being able to accurately and nonjudgmentally sense body sensations helps these patients feel more grounded, centered, and confident and increase their functionality and quality of life. Dan Siegel tells us that studies suggest that people who have more interoceptive abilities "have more capacity for insight and empathy as well as emotional balance and intuition."[2] Developing the interoceptive aspect of Somatic Awareness helps us be better therapists and better people.

Therapist and client observing each other and their environment is "exteroception"—our sensitivity to and our perception of our outside environment. We use our senses of seeing, hearing, touching, smelling, and tasting to get information about the world around us. We receive sensory data through our sense organs and interpret those sensory impressions. We give meaning to this data, which informs our behaviors and attitudes toward ourselves, others, and the world. Therapists use exteroception as a clue to the client's inner system and are aware and cautious of their interpretations, trying to simply notice and stay curious about the meaning of what they observe. Clients use exteroception to gauge their safety, and their perceptions and interpretations guide their behavior.

"Proprioception," another kind of awareness of our internal system considered in Somatic Awareness, uses sensory receptors located in the skin, muscles, and joints that allow us to touch our nose with our eyes closed and walk without looking at our feet. It involves our balance, agility, and coordination. It involves the relationship of our body parts to each other and to the external world. Our proprioceptors give us a sense of our position in space, how we move through the world. They allow us to control the force or effort we move with. We sense tension in our body and the force and direction of that muscular tension. Proprioceptors function largely below our conscious awareness. They can be affected by many factors such as illness, trauma, and aging. Awareness of our muscles, our movement, and our behaviors can help us access our parts, witness their story, and allow the memories in the body's tissues to release, increasing one's proprioceptive capacity. We can bring awareness to the relationship of our body to the space around us and practice new movements and postures, improving our proprioceptive abilities.

I developed all three of these sensory processes in my bodywork training. Studying Structural Integration, I developed my exteroceptive abilities by observing my practice client in stillness and in movement, before and after the bodywork. I learned techniques to address the observed compensatory patterns, imbalances, misalignments, and peculiarities in posture and gait to help my clients move into more ease and wellness. Yet my teacher, Alan Davidson, emphasized that the main goal of this approach was awareness—to increase our client's awareness of their body and their relationship to gravity; in other words, their interoception and proprioception.

This was an important lesson about the essence of a healing relationship. My "fixer" parts took a back seat as I helped my clients connect with the vast network of connective tissue lying just under their skin that encases, supports, and stabilizes all the systems of their body. I developed my sensitivity and my palpation skills as I tuned in to the tissues telling me when they were willing to open to my touch and make a shift, and when I needed to back off. I tracked my client's moment-by-moment response to my touch. I paused frequently to allow my client to notice and to describe what they noticed, both physically and emotionally, to integrate the shifts. My client became an active participant in their healing. Their awareness supported the changes that were available to them. The attentiveness to their body extended beyond my office as they became more conscious of their sensations and postures outside of the sessions.

Understanding that our body is shaped by not only physical but also emotional stresses, I turned to Hakomi therapy to help me address both. Hakomi helped me use exteroception—consciousness of my client's body posture, alignment, and movements—to consider the developmental and psychological issues rather than the structural ones. As a Hakomi therapist I further developed my interoception—my mindfulness of what was happening in my gut and my heart—and helped my clients listen to theirs. I retrained my attention to focus as much on *how* something is said as on *what* is said. Rather than interpretation, I brought curiosity to what I was noting, and I invited my client to engage in a mindful exploration of how their body might be revealing a story of pain or strategies adopted in response to the pain. Together we explored differences between the top and bottom, the left and right, the front and back of their body to open the door to unexplored core beliefs, adaptive strategies, and missing experiences.

With IFS I came to understand the role parts play in interoceptive, exteroceptive, and proprioceptive awareness. Parts' burdens affect awareness, sensitivity, interpretation, and behavior. Perception of the external environment is filtered through parts, and the internal bodymind system processes the information and responds to this incoming data as interoception fuels reactions. Clients' and therapists' parts alike are on the lookout externally for any signs of danger, judgment, and coercion. Much of this data may be below conscious awareness yet driving behavior.

We can be curious about who it is that is seeing, hearing, smelling moment by moment—parts or Self. Burdened parts perceive through the sense organs, and their burdens distort their perceptions and their interpretations of what they have perceived. The burden may dull or heighten both awareness of and sensitivity to the stimuli and induce an escalating cycle of reactivity. For example, the wall color in the therapy office is perceived by the client's part as dangerous, and their internal system is activated. The client notices a racing heart and worries there is something wrong with them. The client's internal system, not finding safety outside or inside, activates their distracting and avoiding parts to cause them to withdraw and numb out. The therapist feels shut out and ineffective. The client hears and sees the therapist's frustration and retreats further. This perception-interpretation-activation behavior cycle might be habitual for this client. Pausing to bring nonjudgmental awareness of the sensations can interrupt this cycle. The conditioned neuronal firing is halted. In the pause created by focused awareness, the burdened part can be invited to see, hear, and sense through the eyes, ears, and senses of Self. Heightening awareness of the parts' mediated responses is an aspect of Somatic Awareness, leading to more choiceful behaviors.

My client Audrey shared her experience as a white woman participating in a gathering of mostly African American social activists as an example of how developing her somatic awareness allowed her parts to step aside. Entering the group she felt tingling in her arms and a warmth in her heart. Then her parts perceived some signs that they interpreted to mean she was not welcome. She felt a wall descend over her heart, an inward pull of her energy, and an opposing impulse to push to be noticed. She brought awareness to these sensations and interpretations and did not act on them. Those sensations diminished and she once again felt energy flowing through her arms and her heart as she moved more freely through the group and contributed to the planning of a protest march.

Our clients who have suffered traumas and wounds of attachment may have disturbances in all of these sensory abilities. These disturbances are symptoms of many psychiatric disorders. Parts of the brain involved in processing the sensory stimuli are either under- or overactive in survivors of trauma. When we are being hurt or mistreated or experiencing sensory information overload, shutting down body awareness is an inherent act largely out of our control, a learned response to regulate our roller coaster of emotions. Developing exteroceptive awareness—to notice approaching footsteps or the smell of alcohol—may have been crucial to survival. Just as hurtful experiences distort and damage our perceptive abilities, the practices of Somatic IFS can safely cultivate these sensory pathways and restore these various modes of perception.

Stephen Porges has coined the term "neuroception" for the ability to perceive neurological safety in the external environment as well as to listen inside the body and between people's nervous systems.[3] His polyvagal theory concerns the action of the autonomic nervous systems to distinguish whether situations or people are safe, dangerous, or life-threatening. When the therapist is in a state of Embodied Self energy, and when the office environment is perceived as a safe place, the client's nervous system is more likely able to move toward the optimal "social engagement" aspect of the parasympathetic state, where there is enough perceived external safety for the client to engage in exploring the inner world. The therapist's nervous system is also potentially activated by perceptions of the client's voice, eye contact, gestures, and postures.

Somatic Awareness Is Associated with the Earth Element

A student of mine discovered the value of the simple act of putting her feet on the ground. "I used to hate to have to wake up. I put it off until the last minute and then I had to rush to get ready and the rest of the day I was not in touch with my body. Then I decided to first put my feet on the ground as I got out of bed. Just to start the day feeling my feet connect with the ground—that has made a difference for me for the rest of the day."

We all need a secure, solid place to stand where we know we belong, just as we are, a place we rest in, a place we move out from. Early relational trauma may have ripped away our connection to a secure, safe sense of belonging. We live in a world with unprecedented challenges—alarming disruptions in our climate, automation and artificial intelligence transforming the workplace, an explosion of technologies, changing norms, personal losses and upheavals. Any time we are startled or afraid, our shoulders automatically hike upward. We feel all of our energy move upward and we lose our ground. We need to find it again and anchor it.

We begin with literally lying, sitting, or standing on the ground or floor. Our first place of grounding was through our navel, while we were in the womb. As we turn and crawl our navel remains a central point we mobilize around as we're extending and flexing our spine, twisting and turning, and learning to coordinate our limbs with our core. The sitting bones of our pelvis become our second place in our body where we connect with the earth. Finally, we venture onto two feet and learn to balance and maneuver as we ground through our feet, exploring the dance of losing and maintaining our balance and our connection. Tuning in to these places, we find the parts that had difficulty with a secure connection. We listen to their body story of fear and abandonment. These parts discover new possibilities for receiving nourishment, for experiencing safe connections, and for finding home base.

All three of these places in our body allow us to connect with energies and qualities from the core of the earth. Even when a client's original attachment to their own mother was blocked in some way, they can connect to the life-sustaining earth energies as these energies enter through the navel, the base chakra (energy center) at the pelvic floor, or the feet. The Latin root *mater* means "mother" and is also the derivation of the English word "matter." We can connect with the archetypal Mother Earth through these places of grounding in our body in addition to all the matter of our body, the densest form of the energies found in our body.

From a secure connection through our body to the earth, we can begin to send out roots, or threads of a web, to find others who share a common ground. This practice of Somatic Awareness links us with others on the planet. We in the United States, connecting with the earth below our feet, may also touch into the question of ownership of the land. Whose land are we standing on? As we connect with the indigenous people whose land we stole, with the animals we have displaced, with a planet becoming overwhelmed by the results of human civilization, we may find in our body a deep sorrow and an apology and a pledge to love better. In the same way as we touch into the earthiness of our body, we uncover dark truths that require our courage, our heartfulness, to embrace and heal.

Body Systems Associated with Somatic Awareness

The Fascial System

Although awareness of our body includes awareness of every system of the body—our bones, blood, nerves, organs—the fascial system is particularly relevant to this practice. The fascial system is the largest system in the body and is the only system that touches every other system, interpenetrating and surrounding them all, enabling them to function in an integrated manner.[4]

Our fascia is central to our awareness of our body in space and our awareness of all that is happening inside our body. This connective tissue literally encircles and encases our whole body, connecting, stabilizing, supporting, and protecting the cells, bones, muscles, organs, brain, nerves, arteries, and veins and the entire body as a unit. The fascial system looks like a spider's web or a densely woven sweater and provides shape, form, and cohesion to the body. It is present just under the skin and in the body's deepest layers. Awareness of this continuous sheath of fibrous, fluid-filled tissue attaching to all these structures in our body, surrounding and linking them into one integrated whole, is the concrete expression of Embodied Self energy. Our parts' burdens that shape our mind also shape our body in the form of fascial restrictions.

The fascia can be considered to be one of our richest sensory organs. It has more sensory nerve endings than our skin. Together with the bones, the fascia facilitates our balance and alignment—our dynamic relationship with gravity, our connection to the earth. The sensory nerve endings embedded within the fascia contribute to both interoception (how we feel inside ourselves) and proprioception (our awareness of our body in space). So when we "go inside" to find out what is happening in our body, it is the interoceptive capacity of the sensory nerves in our fascia that tells us that our stomach is tight, or our jaw or our toes are clenched, or our back is aching. We use proprioception when we notice our posture, balance, and movement relative to gravity. We tune in to our fascia both to listen to our body story and to understand our relationship to our body with our external environment. It links our inside with the outside.

When one client visualized the tension in her body as thick, steel baling wire that was holding all the fragments of her body together, I thought of the fascia connecting, enclosing, and stabilizing muscles and internal organs. As she stayed with the tension and with the connective tissue in her body with a focused, compassionate awareness, it began to loosen and unwind. As she felt her body soften, she discovered an infant part that had been seriously neglected. Without the necessary touch and opportunities for movement, an infant's proprioception does not develop an accurate body map. The nerves become confused about how much effort and force is necessary to stabilize the body. It became clear to this client that the baling wire was trying to bind up this injured infant to keep it from wreaking havoc in her system. As she tended to the infant and to the fragmentation that resulted from her relational trauma, her fascia began to shift. She felt looser yet still held together. Feeling an impulse to move and to dance, she stood up and danced around the room with grace and fluidity while holding the baby.

When our fascia is free, it allows our body to move with grace and strength. When it gets bound up, pain and movement limitations are the result. As a bodyworker I touched into this thin membrane and noticed the places where it was free and the places it was restricted. My clients had described their pain and their limited functioning. My hands felt into the painful adhesions that reinforced and rigidified the dysfunctional ways my clients were using their bodies. My eyes observed how these restrictions affected their functioning. With the appropriate amount of pressure and movement, the glued-together restrictions could be dissolved.

Fascial restrictions have many causes—misuse or overuse of the body, structural and functional issues, frozen emotions. These restrictions and adhesions have many implications for healthcare professionals, but they also have relevance for psychotherapists and other professionals concerned with the bodymind interface. In my practice as a structural bodyworker, it appeared that emotions are held in this web of connective tissue. Touching into my clients' tissues I contacted deep wells of sadness, anger, and fear. It seemed the tissues held memories of failed attempts to escape from overwhelming pain. Bringing awareness through touch and movement released a flood of memories and emotions. Any bodyworker or chiropractor knows the difficulty many clients have in holding their adjustments. I found that when we could integrate the physical with the emotional restrictions and increase the client's body awareness, it made it more possible for the client to sustain the change in both their fascial and their internal family system.

Scientific research on fascia, although still largely ignored, has been focusing on its role in pain, movement, and flexibility. Medical practitioners are now hypothesizing that fascia plays a key role in lower back pain, fibromyalgia, and chronic fatigue syndrome. Several of my colleagues have been considering that the fascia is a communication network for the body. With other bodyworkers I worked alongside acupuncturists in an AIDS clinic in the early days of the epidemic, before the advent of the antiretroviral drugs. Both modalities freed up the flow of energy of the patients and relieved many of their symptoms as well as providing social support. Rather than haphazardly combining structural therapy with traditional Chinese medicine and hoping that our patients might find relief, we practitioners strove to integrate our work. We hypothesized that the fascia might be the connecting link between the Eastern and Western approaches to relieving our patients' debilitating symptoms. We hypothesized that the flow of chi along the meridians travels along this network. Awareness and appreciation of the connective tissue integrated our differing approaches and unified our team. Exploring the connection between our approaches contributed to the realization that we are part of a web of healing cohesive energy that held us all as the virus ravaged precious lives.

When we ignore the messages from our fascia that give us information about how we are, how our parts are, and who we are in each moment and instead distract ourselves with television watching, internet surfing, talking, and analyzing, these sensory nerves are not being exercised. When we practice Somatic Awareness, we go inside to notice what is happening in the depths and interiors of our body. When we practice Somatic Awareness, we notice how we are in relationship to our outside world. When we practice Somatic Awareness, we are awakening the proprioceptive sensory nerves in our fascia that provide us with that information. The practice of Somatic Awareness involves the fascia and strengthens the neural pathways that enable us to both know ourselves and connect with the energies of the wider world beyond our individual selves.

The Central Nervous System

When we listen to our parts speaking through our body, the information from the sensory nerves of the peripheral nervous system embedded in our fascial network is sent to the central nervous system where this input is processed, interpreted, and responded to. When we tune in to what is happening in our body, we engage the ventral medial prefrontal cortex and other parts of the medial prefrontal area. These parts of the brain help regulate the limbic brain and help us be aware of our own feelings and the feelings of others.

According to Daniel Siegel's theory of the mindful brain, awareness of the body builds new neural pathways between the prefrontal cortex and the limbic brain. As he tells us in his book *Aware*, "Where attention goes, neural firing flows and neural connection grows."[5] These new neural connections allow us to have access to the qualities described in IFS as Self energy. He writes of awareness and attention as separate processes that shape the brain and strengthen the mind, and different brain circuits are involved.[6] The practice of Somatic Awareness includes both processes. In Somatic IFS we use brain circuits involved in "awareness" as we find the part in the body, and those involved in "attention" as we focus on the sensations.

The practice of Somatic Awareness not only helps access and locate the part, it also yields greater neural support for Self energy. Trauma in particular disturbs the neural pathways involved in body awareness. Trauma's damaging effects on the nervous system, as well as the path to recovery, are fascinatingly and masterfully laid out by Bessel van der Kolk, one of the premier experts in trauma research and treatment, in *The Body Keeps the Score*. He writes, "Trauma victims cannot recover until they become familiar with and befriend the sensations in their bodies."[7] Remembering the verbal narrative while still being cut off from their physical selves does not lead to a full recovery from the trauma. He believes awareness of the body is the starting point. "Physical self-awareness is the first step in releasing the tyranny of the past."[8]

The road to recovery from the injuries of traumatic wounding begins with the practice of Somatic Awareness. The Somatic IFS therapist helps the client move from dissociation of their body to being able to tolerate their physical sensations and to finally befriending them. The new neural pathways established by Somatic Awareness eventually replace the trauma-related pathways. Somatic Awareness changes the brain.

Our fascial and nervous systems all reveal the interconnected nature of our body. Antonio Damasio sums up the collaborative role of the nervous system in understanding our bodily sensations and therefore our emotions: "These regions and systems participate in the process as an ensemble . . . Once again, those brain regions are not doing it alone; they work in intense cooperation with the body proper."[9] All of our bodymind systems are communicating, cooperating, and collaborating with each other. Each of them is involved in our ability to be aware of our body and in our ability, through this awareness, to help us attain Embodied Self.

Somatic Awareness with a Trauma Survivor

My work with Tanya illustrates how the practice of Somatic Awareness can facilitate every step of IFS. Tanya had a history of trauma and, after seeing many therapists, hoped that a somatic approach could help with her healing.

> Tanya is holding her body tightly as she sits across from me. She sits on the edge of her chair, her head leans forward, her brow is furrowed. I suspect she is also checking me out—and is most likely much better at it than I. Out of necessity, traumatized clients may have overdeveloped their exteroception and perhaps underdeveloped interoception. I want to nonverbally convey a compassionate, confident presence to Tanya so that her "neuroception" is one of safety.
>
> First I focus primarily on my own body. I connect with the places in my body that are touching the chair or the floor. I shift my weight so I am sitting on the sitz bones of my pelvis. I consciously settle my weight into the surfaces below me. With this, my lower body begins to feel denser. Since I know my energy tends to rise up when my thoughts take over, starting the session this way helps me be grounded and connected to my core. I focus on the vertical line between my root chakra and my crown chakra. With my pelvis and spine supporting my head, the back of my neck lengthens. I remind my shoulders they can relax, and the familiar tension in my face can let go. My breath naturally deepens as I focus on it. I breathe into my heart and encourage it to open fully to Tanya sitting across from me.

Finding the Client's Protector Parts

To find a part in IFS, typically we ask, "Where is this part in your body?" But trauma survivors, and other clients whose systems are at risk of dysregulation, may throw up a wall at the therapist's suggestion that they notice what is happening in their body. I will ask a version of this question, such as, "How would it be for your part to let you know how it shows up in your body?" I also will help them identify an area of their body that feels neutral, comfortable, or at least more tolerable to them and ask if they would like to try to be with that place in their body for a short time. However, with Tanya, none of these approaches were appreciated by her protectors.

Although Tanya specifically wanted to work with me because of my somatic approach, her protectors have a different idea. Tanya has spent much of her life alternating between ignoring and controlling her body and being overwhelmed by painful and troubling body symptoms. She had many somatic symptoms that had no obvious physiological basis, such as chronic pain, digestive problems, and insomnia. She realized her trauma was affecting her health and that is why she wanted a somatic approach. But her protectors are not on board with this plan, and they are lining up to defend against this "Somatic IFS."

> One part distracts Tanya, another part didn't hear me and asks me to repeat what I said. Another part makes her so sleepy she can hardly keep her eyes open. Mostly though, she talks. There is a sense she is speaking from a manager part that wants to control the session by talking, possibly to make sure our session would not wander into painful territory. She mostly looks everywhere but at me as she speaks.
>
> I try suggesting, "You might see if focusing on the sensation and letting the story wait for a while helps you to stay present." But she ignores me. I understand that for these protectors, tuning in to the somatic channel risks reliving the horror.

Protectors know that the body stories of the vulnerable parts are stored in the tissues, and they don't want to risk being crushed again by overwhelming sensations. They fear their body sensations will take them down the rabbit hole into oblivion or annihilation with overwhelming sensory flashbacks and the accompanying intrusive, dangerous thoughts and emotions. They want the pain to go away. If they can't get rid of it, at least they can suppress and ignore it. These protectors are fueled by the adaptations in our nervous system that helped us survive for millennia. Our protectors have ready access to a stash of psychopharmaceuticals that they can unleash when they perceive a threat, so it behooves us to not try to oppose these protectors.

Recognizing that for Tanya talking has been a way to regulate and stabilize her emotions, I give her narrating protectors a long leash. They need to know I'm not going to make them change. Her highly developed verbal parts shield her from the fear, shame, disgust, and all the other disturbing emotions and memories trapped in the body. I want to convey compassion rather than condemnation to her parts for their screening capacity. I work with my own impatient part that has an agenda to "do Somatic IFS."

I understand that trauma results in the body, or parts of the body, becoming dissociated, cut off from awareness. As Bessel van der Kolk has noted, "Trauma victims tend to have a negative body image—as far as they are concerned, the less attention they pay to their bodies, and thereby, their internal sensations, the better."[10] Tanya's protectors are determined to shut down her body awareness and to defend against any attempts to get them to do otherwise. I need to remember they have served her well, and, for all I know, their efforts are still vital.

Befriending Protectors

A fitting metaphor for our protective system that helped me develop a relationship with Tanya's protectors is that of a guard dog at a gate, protecting a baby. The dog is there for a good reason, known at first only to the dog. He does his job well, and he will do it unto death. The dog does not trust the stranger who tries to enter the gate to be with the baby. The dog won't be tricked by a pat on the back or a phony bone and will meet force with even greater force. It matters less to the guard dog that the baby is screaming, or lies curled up, frightened and needy, than that the baby be safe from further harm. The guard dog needs to be befriended and appreciated and understood. Then he may permit a glimpse of the baby he is protecting and offer a sense of what he is protecting her from. With this glimpse, the stranger can help the dog change his perception and instead realize this person is a potential helper. The fur on his back lays down, his tail makes a hesitant wag. He sniffs and smells no fear. He looks the person in the eye and is calmed by the kind voice. He now perceives that this person can keep the baby safe and well, and he is free to get his belly scratched or chase a ball.

Gradually Tanya's protectors begin to sense we are truly interested in getting to know them, that we want to hear how they had used her body to protect her from being overwhelmed by her trauma. They had used recreational drugs, smoking, alcohol, and some self-harming behaviors to distract and soothe her pain. Her protectors had alternated between weight gain and loss trying to find safety in her body shape and size. When they realize Tanya and I are listening respectfully to their efforts over the years rather than criticizing them, they begin to relax. When they hear we want to work with them to help the ones they are protecting, they begin to trust us.

Negotiating with Protectors

Tanya's protectors respond well to first being recognized for their efforts before being asked to consider the impact of their behaviors. Relating with the protectors is a delicate, artful dance of respect and recognition for their commitment to their adaptive, decades-old survival strategies while also seeing if they would consider the cost of their efforts—either to themselves or to the system.

The cost is that when we're cut off from our sensate experience, we are cut off from our deepest knowing, from our sensual pleasures, from our relationships with others and the natural world. At our core, we long to regain intimacy with our bodily experience and to explore the intricacies of communication of our tissue, viscera, bone, and fluids. But at first Tanya's protectors were not interested. They said, "It's just the cost of doing business."

Her protectors are willing to consider that perhaps their fears are outdated, that perhaps now it could be possible to let Tanya feel her body sensations for a short while. I let them know I have a lot of experience with this. I invite them to jump back in if at any point they believe Tanya is not safe. As she tunes in to the sensations of her lower body, she feels a "creepy" sensation on her skin. This leads to a part that is disgusted with her softness, her curves, her female genitals. We ask the creepy feelings to dial down so we can stay with them. We stay exclusively with the sensation on her skin. Her protector appreciates that we do not venture into remembering or recounting the painful experience.

Then another protector responds to my invitation to jump back in if it should feel the need. It immediately puts her to sleep. After trying several ways to keep her awake, it is only when I promise to stop this body awareness business that Tanya immediately becomes alert. The part tells us it fears she is becoming "too alive." The part, trying to make sense of the trauma, has attributed blame to her aliveness. When she is alive, she is appealing. When she is appealing, she attracts the attention of her abuser. After feeling understood, this part seems willing to consider that Tanya could notice a body sensation for a few moments. Tanya experiments with brief moments of awareness, keeping in touch with this part. She begins to be able to tolerate, then accept, the array of sensations—temperature, pressure, tension, tingling, even the numbness. Her parts begin to trust that nothing bad would happen.

Working with the Exiled Traumatized Parts

Tanya's vulnerable, traumatized parts are locked behind this band of protectors and are growing increasingly desperate to have their emotions expressed and heard. Emerging from their exile, they are poised to erupt like water from a fire hose, which, of course, would only serve to redeploy her protectors, reinforcing the oscillating cycle of hyper- and hypo-arousal. It is crucial to help Tanya maintain her Self presence so the vulnerable parts will not flood her system in a cathartic re-traumatization, causing us to lose the hard-earned trust of her protectors.

In our sessions, I closely track Tanya's body for signs of emotional dysregulation. I watch for changes in her skin tone, her breathing, her voice tone, pitch, and rate, and changes in her body temperature. I track my own body for signs of feeling a bit dizzy or disconnected from my own body or from Tanya.

As Tanya gets in touch with a three-year-old part and begins to share what she is seeing, I can see she is on the verge of dysregulation. I interrupt the verbal and visual story and direct Tanya to focus solely on the body sensations she is feeling. I ask the part to wait with its story until it can be received. I let Tanya's parts know we want to hear the whole story but we need to slow things down so it can be heard. In this way we slowly reassociate the fragmented traumatic experiences and help all the parts feel held in Self energy.

The body stories emerging from her vulnerable, traumatized parts are often too much for her protectors. Despite my careful tracking, one day Tanya erupts in sobbing, crying out, "I'm a horrible person! I want to die! I should never have been born!" Her body curls up as she holds her stomach with her fists. Her eyes close and her sobbing intensifies in volume and pitch.

I know I need to help Tanya's system downshift. I ask her if she can notice what is happening in her stomach. "It feels icky!" she exclaims. She does not want to stay with this feeling. She is afraid it will get worse. I tell the icky feeling that we can give it a dimmer switch so it can adjust the volume of the feeling. It seems to go along with this notion. The sensations lessen enough that Tanya can focus on it. She feels the urge to vomit. I ask her how she feels toward this urge to vomit, and, reassured the feeling won't become overwhelming, she is able to maintain some degree of curiosity toward it. To help her keep her focus on the sensation, I ask her questions, like where does the ickiness begin and end, what are the boundaries of it like, and what happens to it over time as she stays present to it. The sensations in her stomach lessen as she focuses on them. Tanya's voice and breathing become calmer—lower and slower.

Tanya is able to return to the three-year-old little girl, seeing her, feeling the icky sensations. Tanya feels compassion for her in her warm heart and her tingling arms. She sends these sensations to the little girl, to the icky feeling in her belly. Tanya long suspected she had been molested by her grandfather. Although the three-year-old does not share any images, she sobs, "It's my fault."

Unburdening with Somatic Awareness

Tanya senses the young girl is now sitting on her lap, enfolded in her arms. Tanya tells her that what happened to her was never her fault. It was her grandfather's fault. She tells her she can let go of all the ickiness in her tummy, the belief she should never have been born, the belief the hurt was her own fault. She blows it out of her mouth up into the sky, again and again until she says it is all gone.

Restoring Lost Qualities

After this unburdening, Tanya's stomach feels calm and warm. Her face and eyes are open. Her mouth is relaxed and smiling. She looks at me and laughs with delight. I laugh with her and invite her to stay with the calm, warm feelings in her belly and the sense of this little one in her arms. The little one rests in her lap and Tanya tells her she is so glad to be with her. I encourage her to breathe deeply into her belly, into the space left when she breathed out the "ickiness." Together we enjoy several minutes of breathing deeply, of relaxing together and celebrating that she no longer holds this feeling of being bad and wrong, of her renewed ability to notice sensations in her body, even when they are not pleasant. The unpleasant experiences led her to this precious three-year-old. We are re-storying her trauma as one that no longer needs to keep her cut off from her body to keep her safe, but instead can be a source of safety and stability as well as a trailhead to her exiled parts. This new relationship with her body needs to be reinforced.

Tanya continued to unpack her experiences of being molested by her grandfather. Over time, she was able to focus on her body sensations to keep her emotions from spinning out. Her digestion improved. She quit taking Ambien. She continued to discover sensations, movement, and even touch that she enjoyed. She began to enjoy the soft curves of her body. After exploring this in the safety of our sessions, she began to take her renewed vibrancy outside of our sessions. She enrolled in a salsa class and started dating. She learned to tolerate pleasurable sensations and to ask for the kind of touch that helped her enjoy them. She recovered more of what Joseph Campbell has described as the "rapture of being alive," the birthright of body awareness that is lost with trauma.

After an unburdening, I allow time in the session to notice and anchor the shifts that automatically happen in the client's system. I continue to track the client's physical appearance to notice the spontaneous shifts in their energies, posture, muscle tone, facial expression, and breath. I notice them and name them and invite the client to notice what is different. Many notice changes in their perceptions. Hearing, seeing, touch, or smell may be more vivid. They may notice impulses to move. I understand these are the qualities that got truncated because of the trauma. These moments and even days and weeks after an unburdening are a precious time. Our systems tend to resist change, even positive ones. Parts find safety in familiarity. Without anchoring and integrating the changes into the body and into the behaviors as the client enters their world with several weeks of the new behaviors, the old patterns are likely to reassert themselves. Awareness provides the anchor.

It isn't easy for our parts to reserve ten to fifteen minutes at the end of a session to allow for integrating whatever has shifted, whether or not it is a complete unburdening of a part. I have learned the importance of this time both from my bodywork experience and from yoga. I would notice profound changes to the structure of my bodywork clients as they got off the table. Then they would give a little shake, and look just like they did when they arrived. In yoga the closing posture is *savasanq,* lying on the floor on your back. Yogis will tell us that the ten or so minutes of "doing nothing" are the most important of all the "movements." Yet some in the class seize the moment to check their phones, roll up their mats, and sneak out.

The power of simply bringing our awareness at the end of a session cannot be overstated. My tendency, being a product of Western privileging of doing over being, easily slides toward borrowing a bit of time from the last quadrant of our session to see if maybe just a little more might be accomplished. I am learning, though, the value of reserving at least fifteen minutes to be together with my client with what has shifted. We honor the courage and the parts that showed up and perhaps were willing to trust Self enough to step back. In these minutes we allow time for the unfolding of the changes that began to happen in the third quarter. The spaciousness offers an opening for further flowering of what began to bloom. Perhaps the client shifts from sitting to standing to moving through space to experiment with applying the changes in their world. Perhaps the client notices body sensations when reimaging the original challenging situation described at the beginning of the session. We begin and end the session with Somatic Awareness.

Conclusion

With this practice of Somatic Awareness a secure foundation has been laid for the other practices with every step of IFS. Somatic IFS therapists connect with the earth and their own body awareness as they skillfully navigate the territory of the clients' protectors who believe they need to block awareness of the body. As the protectors learn to trust that attending to the body's sensations as they unfold moment by moment no longer leads to overwhelm and further wounding, they no longer fear awareness. Awareness itself is transformative. The client's sensory abilities are awakened. Their relationship with their body begins to shift. The vulnerable parts whose stories are locked in the body can emerge. The implicit memories and the preverbal attachment trauma are communicated through the body. The therapist not only hears the story but can read the body story being told through posture and facial expressions. The parts' verbal story and body story become one coherent narrative and are fully witnessed by therapist and client. The burdens are released, and the client can more fully inhabit their body. Awareness of their body leads to increased awareness in their body, in every cell and system of the body. Somatic Awareness leads to restoring and cultivating Embodied Self energy.

The practice of Somatic Awareness, shifting from objectifying habits to developing their subjective internal bodily experiences, helps clients rediscover what actually gives them pleasure. By tuning in to their body sensations, they find that exercise and mindful eating are sources of deeper and more lasting gratification than smoking, eating fast food and sweets, and collapsing on the couch to watch television. When the parts that have habitually used substances to comfort, soothe, or smother painful emotions are willing to trust us, we can address the parts they have been protecting—the vulnerable ones holding most of the pain. When the pain held in the body's tissues and organs is released, their bodies come more alive.

Somatic Awareness supports and embraces the other four Somatic IFS practices. We begin with this practice and we weave it throughout the tapestry of the session. Somatic Awareness helps us as therapists be more embodied so we can foster our clients' fuller embodiment. We connect with the earth to bring stability and security to the tumult of the client's inner world. Aware of our fascia, we feel held, supported, and connected. Our sensory nerves assist us in noticing what is inside us and outside us. We help our client tune in to the body sensations of their parts' stories to find healing and release. As the burdens are released, more body awareness is available. Somatic Awareness leads inevitably to the breath, to the second practice, Conscious Breathing.

Now firmly grounded in the solid earth, with this next practice we can feel the energies from above circulating through us. Our vertical alignment is necessary for a Self-led relationship. We rely on our connection with this verticality, our connection with our innermost self, as an anchor in the more complex world of relationship. We return to it when our vertical core of Embodied Self energy begins to feel wobbly from parts that feel uncertain, afraid, or overwhelmed by the energies of another person. When we fully inhabit this vertical line of Self energy through the core of our body, we are the connectors of above and below. As such we have the courage and the resources to enter the subterranean world of our clients with confidence.

EXERCISES

Opening to Somatic Awareness

PURPOSE To establish a baseline in order to keep track of changes. To gauge the level of capacity to tune in to the body and notice sensations and to practice and develop that capacity. To develop the ability to describe sensations in language.

INSTRUCTIONS:

1. If you are new to this, you may want to start with five minutes and gradually increase your time to fifteen minutes. If at any point you begin to feel sleepy or get distracted, just bring your awareness to this. There is no right or wrong way to do this exercise.

2. Lie on the floor. Get as comfortable as possible. Check in with any parts that have concerns about your intention to bring your focused awareness to your body sensations, and see what they need from you and if they are willing to step back. Once they have, you can proceed.

3. Notice where your awareness goes. Does it go to your overall sense of your body? Does it go to areas of pain, or pleasant feelings? Which areas are easier to connect with? Which areas more difficult to feel? Make a map of your body, either imaginary or real, indicating these areas and labeling the sensations.

4. Choose one place in your body to focus on. Stay with the sensation(s) and notice what happens over time with your awareness. Notice how you are feeling toward this place in your body.

REFLECTIONS:

1. What parts were able to step back to allow you to do this exercise? How are they now?

2. Draw an outline of your body, including the words that describe the sensations in the various places in your body, and indicating

the part of your body you focused on. (See the following list of possible sensation words.)

3. How did you feel toward this part of your body? Name it on the body drawing.

4. What effect did your awareness have on this place in your body?

Sensation words: held, numb, tense, irritated, flowing, trembling, cold, warm, heavy, light, tight, loose, calm, burning, aching, moving, dense, still, relaxed, alive, restless, itchy, prickly, blocked

Connecting with the Earth

PURPOSE To experience the sensations of connection with the earth through the feet and the pelvis; to strengthen or restore this connection.

INSTRUCTIONS:

Take a moment of awareness after each of these steps. You might want to do this exercise outside or looking out through a window. This exercise can be done in a fifteen- to thirty-minute meditation, or in a more abbreviated form in between sessions or at the beginning of a session with a client.

1. Stand. Bring your awareness to your feet on the floor or ground. Lift your toes and wiggle them; let them rest down. Lift up on the balls of your feet. Gently bounce on the balls of your feet. Rest your feet. Come up on the balls of your feet again, and let your feet slap back on the ground, several times. Your whole body will jiggle. Do this a few more times. Let the jiggling release unnecessary habitual tensions in the rest of your body. Notice the sensations in your feet.

2. Allow your weight to sink into the lower half of your body. Imagine it slowly sinking like the sands in an hourglass toward your feet. Let your feet meld with the ground.

3. As good stewards recycle what they no longer need, see if there are any tensions, emotions, beliefs, or attitudes you no longer need that you want to send into the earth.

4. Imagine roots from your feet growing down through the layers of earth and rock. Are there particular qualities your parts need that the earth below you can provide? Visualize the roots from your feet absorbing these gifts. Imagine these gifts rising like sap through your body. The marrow of your bones can be the conduit: the bones of your feet, the bones of the legs—tibia, femur—your sacrum, bones of the spine, up to the bones of your head.

5. From the gifts you have received during this meditation, and considering all the gifts the earth has given you since before you were born, notice where you feel gratitude in your body. Send your gratitude from this place downward toward the core of the earth.

6. Come to sitting. Choose a chair that supports vertical alignment, where your hips are slightly higher than your knees and your feet rest on the floor. The floor of your pelvis is also a place of grounding. Invite your pelvic floor to rest down squarely into the seat of your chair and to connect with the earth's energies flowing upward through your bones.

7. Take a few minutes to rest and notice the sensations in your body.

REFLECTIONS   (journal or share with a partner)

1. How does your body feel right now? (sensation words from previous exercise)

2. What thoughts, memories, images, insights, and emotions did you experience during this guided meditation? Do these experiences indicate parts or Self energy?

3. What was released into the earth?

4. What was received from the earth?

5. Did you have any difficulties with any of the steps?

6. Restoring our connection with the earth through our body is said to activate areas of the brain, the autonomic nervous system, the endocrine system, and the immune system. How do you notice any of these shifts?

3

Conscious Breathing:
Integrating Inner and Outer Worlds

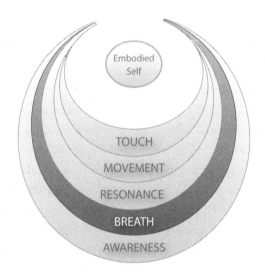

NOTICING OUR BODY, WE become aware of our breathing. Awareness of our breath connects us with the air element, the sky, and the vast cosmos. This second practice of Somatic IFS completes the vertical line begun with Somatic Awareness. Through this vertical line we are connected to above and below. Like a firmly rooted plant we reach for the sun and the stars. We connect with a line of energy from our feet or our pelvic floor through the top of our head and beyond. As the earth is often associated with the feminine element of *being*, while the sky is associated with the male element of *doing*, with this vertical alignment we unite the feminine and the masculine, the being and the doing, the giving and receiving, Heaven and Earth, body and mind, inside and outside. Connected with the ground below, bringing awareness to the air and the space above, we assist the soul's journey embedded in ancient mythologies and contemporary psychologies to marry these seeming polarized qualities and to establish a vertical axis that is our anchor in turbulent times.

At rest, on the average we breathe about one thousand breaths every hour, most of which we are unaware of. Lucky for us, our life doesn't depend on us being conscious of our breathing; it is taken care of by a structure lying deep in our brain stem. Shining the light of consciousness on this largely unconscious act has tremendous potential for assisting the healing process. Bringing consciousness to this involuntary act our life totally depends upon provides a portal to the state of our internal system and to the stories waiting to be revealed.

As I sit with my client and connect with the ground, I begin to be curious about my breath. What sensations do I notice as I breathe in and out? What is the rate of my breathing right now? What places in my body are moving as I breathe in and out? Can I feel the vertical line of energy between the earth and the sky that anchors me? Do I need to make minor shifts in my alignment so this energy can flow freely? I expand my focus to include the space that holds me and my client, the space we are both breathing into and out from. My heart, nestled snugly in between my lungs, opens to my client.

A breath can help my client shift their awareness internally. Some clients find it easier to begin a somatic exploration by noticing their breathing rather than addressing a more general inquiry about their entire body. Protectors and vulnerable parts alike feel held and gently rocked in the rhythms of in and out. Self energy can be sent to parts on the inhale. Burdens can be released through the exhale. New qualities arrive on the inhale. When emotions begin to flood the system, the rhythmic waves of the breath can be an anchor in stormy emotional seas. The therapist can use special breathing techniques to affect an autonomic nervous system that is either highly activated or too sluggish.

A focused awareness of breathing patterns can reveal parts affecting the breath. Bringing awareness to the breath engages various cortical structures, where, along with the kind of awareness we associate with Self energy, we also find the parts that assess our breathing and want to change it. Inasmuch as these protectors can set aside their knowledge of proper breathing, parts deeply embedded in the physical structures of breathing can be revealed. Self energy can be sent to them as easily as breathing. It is never more than a breath away.

Conscious Breathing Is Associated with the Air Element

Awareness of the air element awakens us to our interdependence and the necessity for balanced reciprocity in the exchange of oxygen and carbon dioxide between plants and animals. Every inbreath brings the gift of oxygen released by photosynthesis from our houseplants to the Brazilian rainforest. Every outbreath sends carbon dioxide, the waste product of our cellular respiration, to feed the trees, forests, and fields of swaying grain. Animals and plants need each other to preserve the quality of the air we depend on for our lives. How well we preserve this precious resource will affect living beings for many generations. The rhythm of our breathing echoes this reciprocal relationship. Perhaps the rhythm of taking in and letting go of air can soothe parts that have absorbed toxic burdens from hurtful environments and, perceiving a safer environment, can breathe out what they no longer need.

The element of air also has a metaphysical association and contributes to qualities of Self energy. In alchemy, air carries the spiritual properties to the physical world. In astrology the air element indicates a strong emphasis on mental processes and intellectual pursuits. Air is connected with the light, with our capacity for imagination, for intuition, and for inspiration. As we open to the infinite space above we open to all these potential qualities necessary for our healing relationships.

Connecting with the air element also opens us to receiving gifts from the infinite space around us. Lynne McTaggart, an investigative journalist, has written a paradigm-shifting book claiming that this vibrating space is the ultimate healing force. She describes this field as a vast sea of energy that links everything in the universe in a network of energy exchange.

> There is no "me" and "not-me" duality to our bodies in relation to the universe, but one underlying energy field. This field is responsible for our mind's highest functions, the information source guiding the growth of our bodies . . . The field is the force, rather than germs or genes, that finally determines whether we are healthy or ill, the force which must be tapped in order to heal.[1]

This space that seems like almost nothing might indeed be almost everything. The vastness of this space appears to our senses to be empty, but ever since the birth of quantum mechanics, physicists have known that empty space is not really empty. According to this theory, the space around a particle is filled with countless "virtual" particles. Just as dust motes are revealed by a shaft of sunlight, we learn that nothing contains something. The seeming "void" is seething with energy and particles that flit into and out of existence. The state of *samadhi,* in which the meditator describes feeling a sense of oneness with the universe, reflects the reality of physical phenomena, which at the most fundamental level is primarily empty space. Perhaps this field experienced by meditators and described and studied by McTaggart can be considered in Somatic IFS as the Field of Self energy that surrounds, informs, and nourishes us.

In consultation groups and in trainings, I instruct the participants to listen in a new way to their colleagues sharing a case. We start with a few breaths, consciously letting go of listening habits on the outbreath and opening to a new approach on the inbreath. I ask them to listen not only to the speaker's content but to their own bodies, their internal systems, and to this Field of Self—simply being receptive to whatever information comes to them in thoughts, words, or images. Each participant shares with the speaker the aspects they attended to, and then the speaker responds to all this information that is shared. Quite often, it is the seemingly irrelevant information the participants hear from the field that is most helpful to the therapist sharing their case.

Our body, too, is mostly space. Even though at the level of perception our body is mostly made up of fluid, bone, and tissue, we know that at the subatomic level our body is mostly empty space. About 99.9999 percent is emptiness. Feeling the air touching our skin, breathing in the air, and opening to the space around us, we can experience the spaciousness in our seemingly solid bodies that we often associate with Self energy. When our parts take over, our body feels more condensed than spacious—tight, dense, heavy. Often just a few breaths can open an expansive airiness that makes space for us to differentiate from our parts. The vast sky can hold our parts' pain like a cloud and allow the burdens to dissolve into the atmosphere.

I associate the element of air with the source of guidance that seems to come from without. When I don't know what to do, when I have an agenda, an idea of needing to make something happen *or else,* I open to the space around me, the space holding me and my client. The emptiness of space around me and within me helps me relax into not knowing, into not needing to know. I can open to surprising wisdom from beyond my conscious knowing. IFS acknowledges, in addition to parts and Self, Guides who can assist the Self energy of therapist and client in the process of healing. These Guides appear when welcomed and invited. Sometimes they appear anthropomorphically, while at other times as thoughts or words. In my early days as a therapist I often heard words or thoughts that at first seemed irrelevant or intrusive, and I brushed them aside. But they could be persistent. I learned that their advice was always helpful, and I now trust these voices as wisdom from a source larger than my own, from the infinite space around us.

Conscious Breathing Is a Bridge

Conscious Breathing bridges the practices of Somatic Awareness and Radical Resonance, the intrapersonal with the interpersonal, the unconscious with the conscious, each of us with all other living things and with the spiritual realms. It returns us to the present moment, again and again. When our parts take us into the past with regret and into the future with trepidation, the simple act of noticing our breath brings us back to our body and to the present moment, the only place and time where we can find Self energy.

As a bridge between the unconscious and the conscious, attending to the breath is a valuable tool in psychotherapy. When we bring consciousness to our largely unconscious breathing patterns, we bring awareness to parts that have been lying outside of our conscious awareness. Rapid breathing may point us to a fearful, activated part, while shallow breathing may be associated with dissociation or depression. Differences between the inhale and exhale may relate to existential beliefs, birth trauma, or protective parts trying to control emotions. Sometimes the simple act of bringing conscious awareness to the breath brings a change. A deep, slow breath can be the bridge taking us from anxiety to excited anticipation.

Conscious Breathing is a bridge with all living beings. All humans on this planet, as well as the hawk soaring in the sky, the squirrel scampering through the leaves, the humpback breaching the ocean's surface—all are breathing in and out, depending on the same air. Our mutual need for this life-sustaining gas is perhaps the clearest expression of our unity. Our breathing can expand our consciousness to the transpersonal realms. We become aware that the air surrounding us is the same as the air inside us, and that the Self energy inside us is the same as the Self energy around us. This mutual synergistic exchange of both gas and energy is the universal dance of our essential unity and interdependence.

Our breath links the material and the nonmaterial realms. The connection between breath and Self/Spirit/Soul is evidenced in many cultures and is reflected in their languages. The English word "spirit" is derived from the Latin *spiritus,* which also means breath. The Greek *psyche* means breath and soul; *pneuma* means breath and spirit. The Hebrew *ruah* and Sanskrit *prana* also mean both breath and spirit. *Prana* in Vedantic philosophy is a life force that enters through the breath and travels to all parts of the body. Various breathing techniques, *pranayama,* are a key aspect of the practice of yoga and are used in the practice of Conscious Breathing.

Since ancient times, awareness of the breath has been at the heart of contemplative practices. Through breathing practices one may attain a state of deep consciousness, or *samadhi*. Ideas of the past and the future fall away, and the individual and the universe are mirrors of each other and contain each other. Zen masters liken this state of our mind and body to a clear sky where clouds can arise and pass away. In this state we transcend the illusion of dualism, perhaps our most ubiquitous and pervasive burden. Shunryu Suzuki in *Zen Mind, Beginner's Mind* describes how our breath can lead to unburdening this belief at the core of our suffering:

> When we inhale, the air comes into the inner world. When we exhale, the air goes out to the outer world . . . When your mind is pure and calm enough to follow this movement, there is nothing; no "I," no world, no mind nor body; just a swinging door.[2]

There is a well-known story about a meditator who became bored with the instruction to notice his breathing. When he complained to his teacher that he came to seek enlightenment, not just to endlessly focus on his breathing, his teacher plunged his head into a container of water, releasing him when the act of inhaling could be truly appreciated. Recently a respiratory virus demonstrated very concretely to me how important unrestricted breathing is to our ability to have access to our Embodied Self energy. For two weeks I could not breathe in or out very fully without causing racking coughing fits. I felt literally like I was "beside mySelf" until my bronchials cleared enough for me to breathe fully, and then I had to unlearn the new restricted breathing pattern I had developed during the flu. Like the meditator, I relished the return of the ability to take in and let out full breaths.

A story about the Buddha points to how the simple act of breathing can be a bridge to joy. It has been said that the Buddha disappeared for a month while he was teaching in northern India. Upon his return, his students discovered that he had been on retreat, practicing *anapanasati* (the "full awareness of breathing"). They were perplexed. "Why would you spend time in retreat with such a basic practice when you are already enlightened?" they asked. He replied very simply: "Because it is a wonderful way to live."

The practice of Conscious Breathing bridges what we can control or change and what we cannot. Our breathing, as both a voluntary and an involuntary process, can help us make a shift when it feels like our parts are in control of our moods and our actions. Breath is considered the only voluntary function in the body that can influence the involuntary nervous system. The respiratory system has both voluntary nerves and muscles and involuntary nerves and muscles. The breath can reveal the natural balance of our autonomic nervous system and help us smoothly cross the bridge from activation to relaxation.

The Anatomy of Breathing

To increase our consciousness of our breathing, it helps to know about the physiology of the breathing process and the many different body systems and cell microstructures that collaborate in this largely involuntary act.[3] A more intimate familiarity with the bones, muscles, cells, circulatory system, and nervous system brings the possibility of conscious choice. Consciousness reveals parts and offers a path to return to Self energy.

The journey of the oxygen molecules from the atmosphere to each cell where the mitochondria use it to fuel the cell's life-giving work begins in the brain stem, where a structure called the medulla oblongata automatically detects the levels of carbon dioxide and oxygen in the bloodstream. This primitive brain structure sends nerve impulses to muscles in the diaphragm and is responsible for the involuntary aspect of breathing. If the body needs oxygen, the diaphragm contracts, creating a vacuum inside the chest cavity, drawing in air through the nasal passages. The air travels in through the larynx to the trachea, branches into two bronchi, and enters our lungs. This air is diverted into smaller and smaller microscopic branches, finally reaching tiny sacs called alveoli that diffuse the oxygen molecules through their cell membranes into the capillaries, one red blood cell at a time. When the medulla oblongata detects a buildup of carbon dioxide, that gas is released to the capillaries and travels to the alveoli; the diaphragm muscle relaxes, restoring normal pressure in the chest cavity, forcing air out of the lungs. A healthy adult will repeat this process between ten and twenty times each minute, mostly unconsciously, driven by our primitive brain.

The diaphragm is the major muscular player in breathing. It is a large, thin, dome-shaped muscle that attaches at the lower sternum, at the back to the lower lumbar vertebrae, and at the sides to the seventh through the twelfth ribs. It is like a cathedral ceiling that separates the abdominal cavity containing organs of the digestive system from the thoracic cavity that contains the heart and lungs. When it gets the message from the brain stem that oxygen is needed, this muscle lying above the juicy organs of our belly contracts downward. The dome shape flattens and broadens to resemble a plate as the center moves down, providing a gentle compression of the organs below. As the diaphragm pushes down, the edges lift up, causing the thoracic cavity above to expand, drawing air into the lungs. When the diaphragm relaxes and returns to its original dome shape, the elastic recoil of the thoracic wall causes this area to contract, forcing air out of the lungs. Other muscles of the neck and thoracic area are also involved in the action of breathing. The respiratory diaphragm shares a relationship with the pelvic diaphragm as well as the soft palate of the mouth. All these muscles are attached to and interact with our bones—the ribs, the sternum, the clavicles, the spine, and the cranial and pelvic bones.

Our autonomic nervous system (ANS) is another major system involved in breathing. When we inhale, we activate the sympathetic branch of the nervous system (SNS), which has been likened to a physiological gas pedal that activates us to respond to a perceived threat. When we exhale, the parasympathetic branch (PNS), likened to the brakes in our car, inhibits the sympathetic branch. The SNS quickens our breath, the PNS slows it. According to polyvagal theory, when we perceive danger our SNS is mobilized to fight or flee. If we successfully return to safety, a more evolutionarily recent aspect of the PNS puts a brake on our sympathetic activation, and we feel calm and safe. If we are not successful, a more primitive part of our PNS takes over, and we shut down, collapse, dissociate. The breathing pattern may be fixed in the rapid, high breath of SNS mobilization or the slower, shallow breath of PNS dissociation, or it may oscillate wildly between these two extremes.

Our parts can cause our ANS to keep its foot on the gas, or even press on the gas and the brake at the same time, wearing out our systems in the same way our car would quickly wear out. When controlled by a conscious process, though, breathing can regulate the gas and brake pedals of our ANS as well as our pulse, blood pressure, digestion, and metabolism. Breath can be the pathway from the dissociated PNS state to the mobilized SNS activation and finally to the more evolved PNS state of social engagement for both client and therapist.

Fostering Consciousness of Breath

Bringing awareness to the anatomical structures involved in breathing expands consciousness of the breathing process, providing a gateway to parts in our internal system and a path to Embodied Self. We can notice the degree of movement of our rib cage—my German translators tell me that the exact translation of the English "rib cage" is "rib *basket*." Bringing touch and awareness to this flexible basket of bone and muscle that the respiratory muscles attach to—front, sides, and back—may help the thoracic area soften, allowing for a fuller inhale and a more complete exhale. The ribs attach to the sternum in the front. Placing a hand on the sternum as we inhale, we feel the upward and outward motion of this bone. Moving our hand to the area just below our sternum, our hand moves outward on the inhale and inward on the exhale. Our collarbones (clavicles) and all the attached bones and muscles of our shoulders and arms float above the rib basket. With our other hand on our stomach, we feel the rhythmic expansion and condensing in our belly. Moving this lower hand to our back, we feel the diaphragm flattening out as the breath moves in and out of our body. Moving our hands to the sides of our ribs, we follow the action of the diaphragm and the intercostal muscles raising and lowering the rib basket. With a hand under the pit of each arm we feel the upper lobes of the lungs filling up and emptying with air.

Awareness of these movements may immediately result in a fuller range of movements and a change in our breathing. We might notice subtle movements in our head and neck, shoulders and arms, spine and pelvic floor.

Our breath may become slower, deeper, fuller. Along with the changes in our breathing, we might experience an increase in some of the qualities of Self energy. We might find, as the Buddha did, that attending to our breath is a wonderful way to live. Or we may be becoming more conscious of restrictions in our breathing, or, like the beginning meditator, we may feel bored with focusing on this simple act.

For many people, bringing awareness to the act of breathing can trigger parts. Consciousness of breathing patterns can activate existential issues related to attitudes toward life and death. Listening to our breath can reveal our stories embedded in our nervous systems. Trauma survivors can become overwhelmed by focusing on their breath, so it is important to consider the role of the autonomic nervous system with breathing.

My friend and colleague Deb Dana has recently expanded my appreciation of the practice of Conscious Breathing as it relates to the ANS. Her book *The Polyvagal Theory in Therapy* describes her method of tracking, noticing, and naming our breathing patterns in order to assess the state of our ANS as well as to regulate and shape it by befriending the flow of our ANS. Once the particular ANS state is recognized, Dana suggests some breathing practices to shape the state of nervous system activity to provide a repair and an experience of relational connection and safety:

> Generally, slower breathing, prolonged exhalations, and resistance breathing increase parasympathetic activity. Matching inhalation and exhalation maintains autonomic balance, while rapid breathing, irregular breathing, and sharp inhalation or exhalation increase sympathetic activity.[4]

Consciousness of our breathing allows us as therapists to assess the state of our ANS and to shape it so that we can provide a safe connection for our clients to notice and shape their ANS. Through this process of co-regulation of our ANS, burdened parts are welcomed into an atmosphere of safety and trust where their stories can be seen and told. Clients and therapists can recognize how their breathing is related to their physiological state, and how their physiological state creates a psychological story.

When attention to the act of breathing signals danger, there are many breathing practices that can shift the client's ANS so that they can bring the energy of a safe and compassionate connection to the parts telling their stories. The balanced breathing Dana mentions, known as four-square breathing, can be a way to safely introduce breathing practices as well as to manage anxiety. Yogic breathing such as the breath of fire or the breath of joy can bring in more energy to a collapsed, frozen state. The client can experiment with gradually increasing either the exhalation or the inhalation to see which brings them the most comfort, relief, and safety. Dana also suggests bringing attention to the exhale, to the automatic sighs that accompany the exhales of her clients, as a way to acknowledge the inherent wisdom of their autonomic nervous systems working to bring regulation to their systems. Similarly, I encourage yawning on the inhale as well as sighing and sounding on the exhale as a way to shift the ANS from sympathetic activation to the parasympathetic ventral vagal state.

Just as conscious awareness of our breathing can access parts, intentional breathing practices can help us differentiate from parts and bring Self energy to them through the breath. Just as yogis believe the breath carries *prana* up the spine and to any place in the body, in the practice of Conscious Breathing we can send Self energy with our breath to anywhere in our body, no matter how far from the lungs. We find a quality of Self, such as curiosity or compassion, and breathe into that place. The breath can awaken and enliven the flow of Self energy, and from there we direct the breath to any place in our body.

Embodied Speech in Somatic IFS

When the parts need to tell their stories, Conscious Breathing can help the parts give voice to their pain. Often parts were burdened before they could communicate about their feelings and needs. Their truths may not have been allowed to be given voice. They may not have been listened to or believed. Their pain may be cut off, buried in tissues. Words may not be able to find the places where they are buried. Other parts may attempt to tell the stories. The verbal telling feels disconnected from the place in the body that the words are born from. The truth that is wanting to be known fully is trapped in the muscles and organs involved in breathing and in speech, causing the voice to sound artificial, strained, flat, or hushed. The stories have not yet found a way to be told in embodied speech. Sometimes before the truth is born, before it becomes words, it begins as a sound, a sigh. The sigh may be the first whisper of something hidden inside, something waiting to be born, waiting to become a word. An exhale can lead to a sigh, which leads to the sounds and the words connected to our truth, which allows our speech to be embodied.

One breathing technique from yoga can help the client begin to find their voice. In this technique, called *ujjayi* breath, on the outbreath the muscles of the larynx are contracted, adding resistance to the exhalation. The sound that the exhale makes is like the waves of the ocean, so it is sometimes called ocean breath. This breathing practice accords many physical, emotional, and spiritual benefits. It increases the oxygen in the blood, builds internal heat, cleans out toxins, and improves the immune system. The vibrations in the larynx stimulate the sensory receptors that signal the parasympathetic nervous system to slow the heart rate and lower blood pressure. *Ujjayi* breath can bring many qualities we associate with Embodied Self energy, such as calm, confidence, and clarity. It also can open the door for the client to find her voice, as it did with my client Judy.

Judy feels shaky. Her breath is shallow. She says it feels like something in her chest is bracing her against an enemy. I suggest she try this ocean breath, noticing the sound. For several breaths I guide her to take in only as much breath as feels OK to her and to breathe out with this ocean breath, listening to the sound. She becomes comfortable with the sound of her outbreath and even feels comforted by it.

After several breaths, her shakiness lessens. Her inbreath is easier and fuller. She continues to listen to the sound of her breathing, and soon the sound becomes a sigh. At first the sighs are sighs of relief that the fear and the tension reduced. Then she says the sighs change to feelings of sadness that lay underneath the fear.

As Judy stays with the sadness that emerged, she feels some tears behind her eyes that can not come out. I ask her to tune in to the place in the body where the sad sigh originates. I ask her if she can hear the sound the sad part is making inside. When she says she isn't sure, I suggest she try some different sounds. When she seems to feel a bit self-conscious, I softly join her as she experiments with various vowel sounds and different pitches. We try "aaaahhh" and "oooohhh." We make these sounds in different pitches and volumes. Finally a soft, highly pitched "Ooouuu" comes out of Judy's mouth, bringing the tears the part was wanting to shed.

Through breathing, sighing, and sounding, Judy is freeing up the voice of her vulnerable parts to express their story and their emotions.

Parts affect voice quality—the timbre, tone, intonation, rhythm, pitch, pace—and parts-led speech or embodied speech is evident from these differences. When I speak with my clients by phone I listen to the timbre, tone, and pace of the voice to assess the state of their body and their nervous system. Susan Aposhyan, who has integrated Body-Mind Centering with psychotherapy to create Body-Mind Psychotherapy, writes that the work of freeing up our innate tendency to vocally express ourselves is often neglected in therapy:

> As human beings have worked to hide their internal process from others, we have habituated a tendency to repress our vocal expression. Rather than sighing, groaning, grunting, yelling, crying, or laughing, we run all our vocal impulses through a neurological mechanism to censor these for social acceptability.[5]

These vocal expressions are literally the soundtrack of the body stories. Many people have been shamed or punished for loud speech, angry speech, and screaming, and the protector parts have had to be the censors. Certain words may have been taboo. Sometimes in a session the inhibiting protectors are overridden and the sounds or words are uttered spontaneously. The vocal expression of the exiled part needs to be welcomed and encouraged while the protectors are reassured. Bringing awareness to the sound and mindfully repeating it can open a pathway to healing.

IFS is not a catharsis model. The point is not to purge emotions but to restore voice to the silenced, exiled parts and have them be heard by

Self. Many people will only cry silently. It may be possible for words to be spoken, but the authentic emotions are absent from the content. An angry message may be conveyed with a tone of sweetness or couched in an apology. Embodying speech may start with first hearing internally the words "I hate you!" We notice how the body responds to the sound. We then ask if the parts are OK with having the client say the words or make the sound that they hear inside. This process can be profoundly empowering to parts that have been silenced and shamed. We find where the words originate in the body. With permission from the protectors, we allow the sound to ride on the wave of the outbreath, supported by the core musculature.

Parts reveal themselves through the voice. As we listen to our clients talking, we note the voice quality as well as the content. The voice quality might change, suggesting another part just showed up. We may hear the voice of a child. We can ask the client, "Who is it that is talking right now?"

In my session with Alex I was struck by the tone of his voice as he reassured his young part that what happened to him was not his fault. His words were good, but his voice was not reassuring. It was high, tight, and shaky. It seemed like his little-boy part was blended with his body—at least with his vocal cords. I wondered how to help Alex speak from his Embodied Self rather than from the scared little boy. I asked a question to determine his access to this energy.

SM: How do you feel toward this little guy, Alex?
Alex: I feel bad for him. I guess it is compassion.

The tone and words both suggested he wasn't there yet, but I thought we could build on it.

SM: Where do you feel this compassion in your body?
Alex: In my heart.
SM: Breathe into your heart. Let your outbreath carry the compassion from your heart to your throat. Let your words come from your heart.

After several breaths Alex's voice became slower, lower pitched, and more resonant as he told the little boy that none of it was his fault.

The therapist's embodied speech conveys the presence of Embodied Self energy and is more important than the words that are spoken. The therapist's voice is like a musical instrument that shifts the internal state of the client. A slower, softer tone can support the client to slow down and go inside. The pitch of the voice influences the autonomic state. Polyvagal theory tells us that speech that is too low in frequency can signal the presence of predators, while monotones and high pitches convey pain and danger. Prosody, which includes intonation, tone, pitch, and the rhythm of speech, can be either a cue to danger or an invitation into the safety of the ventral vagal state of social engagement.

A therapist can ask the client a question with a pitch and timbre that conveys either openness or interrogation, compassion or judgment. Nothing reveals our parts like the tone of our voice. We may not be aware of our tone when we speak. We can track our clients to gauge whether the tone, pitch, volume, and rhythm of our speech is inviting the ventral vagal state of social engagement or perhaps is activating the ANS arousal of their parts. I have become aware that my pace can speed up when a part is concerned about time. When I don't feel understood I get louder, and probably convey frustration. Bringing my breath to my lower belly and allowing that to support my voice can help get me back on the track of Embodied Speech.

The Practice of Conscious Breathing in Somatic IFS

Sufi mystic and poet Rumi has written about breathing: "There is one way of breathing that is full of shame and constriction. Then there is another way: a breath of love that takes you all the way to infinity." Somatic IFS addresses both ways of breathing noted by Rumi. For the most part I simply bring awareness to the breath. Noting the constrictions, disruptions, and irregularities in breathing patterns, we may access parts with burdens of shame, fear, sadness, despair, or rage. I also employ "the breath of love"—particular breathing techniques that take my client, if not all the way to infinity, perhaps toward a bit more Embodied Self energy as the autonomic nervous system is more under vagal control.

Conscious Breathing Assists the Therapeutic Relationship

The process of IFS therapy, and of course Somatic IFS therapy, begins with the therapist in as pure a state of Embodied Self energy as their parts will allow. Our breathing pattern can reveal our degree of Self energy, and changing it can increase it.

As I meet with my client Kevin for the first time, I notice my breath is a bit rapid. So is my heartbeat. Clearly a part of me is anxious. I breathe deeper into my abdomen with my inhale, bringing more awareness to my lower belly. I breathe out more slowly on my exhale. I feel more spaciousness in my torso. I feel more open, not just inside my body, but also it seems like my awareness is more open. I become aware of the space around me and Kevin. I inhale this energy into my heart. I feel curious about what has brought Kevin and me together. Within the space of a breath or two, my heart rate and my breath slow down. I consciously breathe out energy from my heart into the space around me and my client Kevin.

Kevin quickly spills out the problems he hopes I can help him with. As Kevin is speaking, I notice tension in his jaw. I watch the rise and fall of his chest and abdomen. Most of the movement is in his upper chest with some restriction in his lower torso. His breath is faster than mine is now. For a few breaths I mirror his breathing pattern to increase my resonance with him. I wonder if a part of him is anxious. I wonder if it is related to what he is talking about or if this is his breathing habit. I return to my own breathing pattern for a breath or two. I then breathe in his anxiety and breathe out the energy from my heart. I remind myself to check in with my breathing during the session.

Conscious Breathing Helps the Client Go Inside

Once Kevin and I have a sense of the focus for our session, I direct his attention to turn inward to explore his inner world. Kevin has difficulty with this shift. I wonder if he assumed that the process of change, based on his work with his last therapist, occurs through his conveying data for me to sort out and offer interpretations and guidance. It is also possible that he, like many others, has found that talking and focusing outward has kept him from being swallowed up by overwhelming feelings, and perhaps it has become a habitual protection.

My diaphragm tightens with the thought that maybe Kevin and I are not a good fit. With a breath into my lower abdomen, my stomach loosens up. I feel curious to get to know this person in front of me. I am wondering how I can help him without getting pulled into being his fixer. I explain to Kevin how I work and ask him if he would be willing to let me help him turn his attention inward to find his parts involved in these problems. He is willing.

SM: Your parts connected with these problems might show up first as feelings, words, images, or body sensations. You can start by noticing your breath. You don't need to breathe any particular way. Just pay attention to your breath going in and coming out.
Kevin: [*laughing*] What breath?
SM: Right. Let's start with the sensations in your nostrils as the air comes in and goes out. Now notice any movement in your chest. Place your hands on your ribs.
Kevin: My breath is not very deep.
SM: See if you can let go of the tension in your jaw, and just keep noticing that you are breathing in and breathing out.

I see he is still breathing quite shallow and fast.

SM: Try to take a little pause at the end of your exhale.

Kevin looks at me with some skepticism, but when this allows his breath to become a little slower and deeper, he feels calmer and looks at me with a bit more trust in his eyes. He closes his eyes and is willing to listen inside to find what he wants to focus on in our session.

Conscious Breathing Accesses Parts

A whole world of parts can be accessed simply by observing the pace, flow, and rhythm of breathing patterns. Manager parts have learned to control feelings by tightening the muscles and fascia of the torso and diaphragm as well as the mouth and jaw. Posture is affected as the chest tightens or collapses, and the fixed posture in turn prevents fuller breathing. Other manager parts may have learned "correct" breathing patterns that overlay these earlier protective patterns, replacing the parts' induced restricted breathing with compensated deep breathing. Another category of protectors, the "firefighters" react when they perceive that danger is present, internally or externally. Their breathing patterns may resemble either that of rapid, shallow SNS activation or the dissociated PNS activation. Belief systems are revealed in habitual breathing patterns. Parts that restrict the inhale may believe they don't deserve to receive. Parts that restrict the exhale may have fears of letting go, fear of dying, or a deep desire to give up and never breathe in again.

One of the issues Kevin wants to explore is his addiction to cigarettes. As he recognizes the pleasures of deep breathing, he is realizing how much he needs the comfort and relaxation his inhale gives him, and that smoking allows him to breathe deeply. He commits to pausing when he feels the impulse to light up, and during that pause to practice deep, full inhales. This allows him the space to choose whether to smoke or to continue to breathe without the smoking.

There are many moments during the day when Kevin reaches for his pack and lights up without the breathing practice. But gradually he finds the breathing helps him cut back. This is his first step toward quitting smoking. He begins to enjoy the calm that comes with the deep, slow breathing. He also notices how automatically his habitual rapid, shallow breathing takes over.

Kevin brings his awareness to his breathing pattern. He notices some tension in his stomach when he inhales, which eases when he takes shorter, shallower breaths. He is curious, so he breathes into the place of tension to see what is there. He is surprised to find a timid young boy about ten years old. He begins to tell me that he was often bullied growing up. His schoolmates taunted him for being gay before he even knew it. He told no one about it, afraid he somehow deserved it. As he begins to share with me about one particular experience being bullied on his way home from school, Kevin starts to get agitated. His breath comes faster and his eyes begin to dart around the room.

When Parts Take Over

Many beginning IFS therapists struggle when their clients' parts (or their own!) seem to be sucking any Self energy out of the room. There are many reasons our parts believe they need to take over. Sometimes protectors are making sure the vulnerable parts stay exiled. They can muster tremendous amounts of power and control, as well as ingenious creativity, if they believe it is for the benefit of the system. They don't trust the Self. They think the Self is another part that is going to overpower them. It never works to trick them or argue with them or coerce them. Vulnerable parts can also flood the system with their emotions. They believe they have two choices—either a total takeover to make sure they will be heard and helped, or being locked up again where they are isolated and hopeless.

When Kevin's exiled experience of being bullied begins to surface, the emotional and physical expression erupts so powerfully that he cannot be present to the vulnerable young boy. The part is blended, and it floods his system with all the physiological signs of SNS activation.

I am glad the young boy has emerged and I want him and his painful story to be met with Self energy—Kevin's as well as mine. I notice a slight echo of SNS activation in my body as well. I tune in to my diaphragm, let out a long breath, and decide to direct Kevin to focus on his outbreath to help his exile unblend. I intentionally calm my voice.

SM: Let's drop the story for now and return to your breath. Focus on the outbreath. As you breathe out, purse your lips like you do when you breathe out cigarette smoke. Breathe it out slowly and completely. Just focus on the exhale.

I did this pursed-lips breathing together with Kevin for several breaths.

SM: What are you noticing now about your breath and your stomach?
Kevin: It seems like the long exhales help slow my breathing. I am breathing more into my abdomen. I feel calmer.

Kevin's trauma was frozen in his respiratory muscles from his jaw down to his diaphragm, controlling his breathing patterns. He finds breathing—both attending to his natural breathing as well as particular breathing techniques—to be an effective practice to navigate the cycle of hyper- and hypo-arousal connected with his trauma.

With his emotions regulated and his safe connection with me restored, he is now able to bring this Self energy to his young part with the story of being assaulted and taunted by several boys on his way home from school. The young boy feels comforted by his presence and relieved to have his painful story brought out in the open. His burden of isolation and fear seems to dissolve as this part feels connected with Kevin.

Conscious Breathing with Unburdening

Kevin's young part had absorbed the burden that the abuse was his fault. His part believed he must be bad to deserve such treatment. Other boys were not getting beat up, but he was. Being bad was associated with being gay. Growing up in our homophobic society, he suffered with this burden throughout his life, especially when some members of his family could not accept his sexual orientation.

Kevin's part tells us it wants to let go of this belief that he is bad. He finds the burden as a clenching in his stomach and his abdomen. When I ask Kevin how he would like to begin to let go of this badness, he rises from his chair, and standing with his legs apart, closes his eyes and makes a fist.

Kevin: [*yelling*] Stop it! Leave me the fuck alone! [*He breathes out huge puffs of air.*] The badness is coming out through my breath.
SM: Keep going. You are doing great. Let go of all of it.

Kevin rests for a moment, then continues with more stomping and yelling. As he seems connected with his Self, I encourage him to let all this badness out of his body.

> Kevin: [*voice slightly lower*] Get out of my body. If you won't accept me, that's your problem!
> SM: All of that clenching in your body, all that badness, let it go out with your stomping, your words, your breath.
>
> Kevin breathes out in great gasps, fully exhaling. His breathing gradually slows. His face looks relaxed, his chest seems fuller. He tells me he feels like there is a vibrating motor turned on in his body. I encourage him to stay with the feelings of vibration and move around the room, enjoying the sense of breathing in a world where it is fine to be gay.

Because there are places and people where it is not yet safe to be gay, Kevin has found that when situations in his present life activate him, he can focus on his breathing as a way to calm himself. It is a comfort to him that calmness could be a breath or two away.

Case Examples with Conscious Breathing
Making Space for Unresolved Grief

My client Naomi is committed to her practices of yoga and meditation. She had noticed during her meditation and her pranayama practice that her exhale was more difficult for her than her inhale, and she wanted to use our session to find out about it.

> Naomi focuses the act of her breathing and immediately finds a part that judges her breathing and wants to change it. It willingly steps aside. She now is just curious. She feels the expansion in the middle of her lungs on the inhale, and notices a restriction as the breath leaves. She studies the restriction. She finds some tension in her navel. At that, a feeling of sadness begins to rise up toward her throat. The tension grips her navel area more strongly, but Naomi stays calm and curious toward the sadness and the tension.

SM: Breathe into this tightness at your navel. Like your breath is saying a gentle hello.

Naomi: The tension is holding back the sadness. It thinks we are going to try to make it let go and then the sadness will be too much. It will engulf me.

SM: Let it know we are on its side. We don't want you to be engulfed by sadness. We understand it has been important to keep the sadness down because it would have been too much for you to feel. Send this message on your breath as you breathe into the tension.

Naomi: My exhale can be a little deeper now. I feel a little sadness coming up but so far it isn't too much for me.

SM: Where in your body is this part that feels sad?

Naomi: It's here, in my second chakra. I am sensing a young girl. She's about seven. She is crying. She misses Daddy. After my parents' divorce, he moved away and started another family. I didn't see him much after that.

Naomi breathes into her stomach, sending welcome and love to this little girl on the inhale. She invites her to share her sadness on the exhale. Naomi continues in this way for many more breaths, shedding some tears, breathing more deeply, and feeling calmer. She decides to continue this relationship through breathing in her meditations.

Breath and Sound to Heal Sexual Wounds

Martha, a rape survivor, was having difficulties with her sexual relationship. Newly married for the second time, she had been avoiding her husband and was afraid her unresolved trauma would ruin this relationship.

We decide to start with the part that is afraid of being sexual with her husband. As she tells me about some recent failed attempts to be intimate with him, I notice her breathing is rapid and shallow.

Martha: [*in a tight voice*] I'm afraid of him.

SM: Does it feel right to say "a part of you is afraid of him"?

Martha: Yes, it helps to remember it is just a part of me.

SM: Where do you notice this fearful part in your body?

Martha: It's all through my core. I also can tell I'm not breathing very deeply.

SM: Let's see if it helps to bring a breath into the core of your body, letting your breath touch the places that are keeping your breath shallow, and notice if the part is willing to speak with you about its fear.

Martha: This is the thirteen-year-old. She thinks all men are dangerous. She is afraid that if she gave up her fear she would turn into a little puddle and she could be raped again.

Martha's breathing again becomes more rapid, shallow, and confined to her upper chest. I ask the part to wait to tell more of its story while she and I attend to her breathing. On the inbreath Martha lets her thirteen-year-old part know she is with her. She consciously breathes out long, slow breaths, telling her part she is safe now.

Martha: Now I see a girl who wants to run away. But I will ask that part to step back.

SM: Before you do that, ask the part that wants to run away if it is her, the thirteen-year-old.

When Martha says yes, I tell her to encourage this girl to run to a safe place. She runs to Martha's backyard. Martha is there with her and together they notice the sights, sounds, and smells in her backyard.

SM: What is happening now in the core of your body, with your breathing?

Martha: My core is feeling cool and spacious, filled with white light. But my shoulders are still tense. It's still hard for me to breathe.

SM: Just stay with your breath, noticing both what makes it hard and the sensations of breathing in and out, the movements you notice. Breathe into the cool, white, spacious core, and purse your lips as you breathe out. As your breath travels past your larynx, see if you want to make a sound. Maybe you hear a tone, or a vowel sound that you would like to make as the air vibrates through the larynx.

At first the sound Martha makes is rough and gravelly, but as she continues experimenting with different tones and vowel sounds, she tells me she enjoys the vibration in her sternum and in her shoulders. For several minutes she alternates the sounds with the pursed-lips breathing. She tells me the girl likes the sounds too. Martha's shoulders relax. Martha asks the girl if she could let go of all her fear now that she is in a safe place. She releases her fear to the universe.

After this unburdening, Martha asks her if she is still afraid to have sex with her husband. The girl says that man hurt her, but her husband has never tried to hurt her. Martha tells her part that when they have sex, it is not the thirteen-year-old he is having sex with, but the grown-up Martha who is having sex. Martha tells me the girl relaxes when she hears this, and she notices her shoulders are even more relaxed and she can breathe more easily.

Transforming Anger through Breath and Sound

Sophia was a participant in a Somatic IFS three-day seminar. She volunteered to be the client in front of the group in order to demonstrate Somatic IFS. As I sat before her, all of us took a moment to connect with the earth and with the space around us. We closed our eyes and breathed into our hearts, setting the intention to hold Sophia in Self energy.

When I open my eyes, I see that Sophia is very activated. Her hands are held tightly in her lap, her breath is rapid and shallow.

SM: OK, Sophia. I see there is something happening in your body. Would it be OK to start with this?

Sophia: There is a band of tension [*pointing to it*] from the back of my neck to the throat.

SM: How do you feel toward this tension?

Sophia: I would like to find out about it.

SM: OK, you could ask the tension what it is afraid would happen if it were not here.

Sophia: I would be in a rage.

SM: Can it show us or tell us what is dangerous about your rage?

Sophia: [*laughing*] I might flatten somebody.

SM: Was there a time when you did flatten somebody?

I am surprised by her reaction. Sophia shakes her head yes and begins to get even more agitated. She blows her nose and rapidly rolls out a story about how she came home and found her father, drunk again, lying on the front steps to the house, and she said some very mean things to him. I know I need to slow the process down or her system will soon be completely flooded with the emotion that is eager to explode.

SM: I want to hear the rest of the story, but right now I want you to pause and notice what is happening in your body as you have been talking.
Sophia: Now I feel more tension, like a collar around my neck and shoulders. It is hard to breathe. It is hard to move my body at all. I feel frozen.

I can see this tension in her body. Her neck and shoulders look like the lid of a pressure cooker, and I sense the energy from below wanting to erupt. I don't need to ask how she feels toward this tension. I can tell she has little available Self energy—she is beginning to get flooded emotionally and physically, and she is driven by a strong impulse to continue with the story.

SM: Look into my eyes for a moment. How is it now?
Sophia: It calms down a little.
SM: Good. Let's go for a bit more calmness. Do you remember that we talked about breathing through pursed lips to help calm down our nervous system? Can you do this now while you look at me?

As Sophia does this, I can see some calmness restored. I ask her how old she was when she found her father drunk. She tells me she was eighteen. Sophia leaps back into the story.

Sophia: That day it was like the last straw. I jumped over his body, said some very nasty thing to him, and then spit on him.

I tell Sophia it is important for her to really resonate with the story as the eighteen-year-old is telling it. I want Sophia to be able to be present with her part that holds the strong feelings so she can help her digest this clearly overwhelming story.

SM: Can you ask the eighteen-year-old if it is OK if at times I ask her to pause her story so she can stay more calm?

Sophia: Yes, she is glad to have your help.

SM: Let's rewind the tape on this story and go back to when you had the impulse to jump over his body on the front steps. Where do you feel that impulse?

Sophia: It's right here. [*pressing her hand hard into her diaphragm*] It's like a stone.

SM: Good. Stay with that stone. Focus on it. Let your breath touch it. Let it know you understand this was the last straw.

Sophia: Yes, it is softening. It doesn't feel like a stone anymore.

I am about to suggest we retrieve the eighteen-year-old and bring her into the present, helping her unburden these strong emotions.

Sophia: And then he died.

I feel the shock go through my body. I let it go out my breath. I re-establish my vertical connection. I then ask her to look into my eyes again.

SM: Sophia, would you like if we could redo that awful day when your rage erupted at your father? [*When she says yes, I continue.*] OK, we will both go into that scene to be with her.

Sophia sits on the front steps of her house in between her father lying prone on the steps and the eighteen-year-old. I am with her too. Her part tells us she never got to have a childhood.

SM: How would she like things to be different?

Sophia: She would like me to speak to him for her even though he may not be able to hear it.

Sophia begins to speak in a low, controlled voice to her father about his mistakes, her anger, and her sadness of the loss of her childhood. She tells him he made many, many mistakes. Her voice seems constrained as she says these words. I ask her to feel where her anger originates, and she again points to her diaphragm.

SM: Breathe deeply into that place where you find the anger. Let your voice come from there as you say, "You made many mistakes."

This time her voice is clear, strong, and deep. Her spine length-ens. I sense there may be more that could be expressed if we were not so focused on the words.

SM: Breathe again into this anger, and on the exhale just make a sound that expresses that anger.

She tries several different tones and vowels. She breathes into the sadness about not having a childhood and breathes out a differ-ent sound. Sophia's appearance changes. She now looks calm and happy. She looks powerful.

Sophia: You know, I feel love for my father. Even though some people don't want me to love him, I still do.
SM: Yes, I'm glad you can feel that. Breathe into this place where you feel the love and speak from that place.

Sophia tells her father that she loves him. She tells me that express-ing her love was a vital missing experience in her final moments with her father. As the session comes to a close, she says the tension in her neck, throat, shoulders, and stomach is completely gone. She feels free and loving.

Conscious Breathing Leads Us to the Practice of Radical Resonance

Breathing, as a bridge in so many ways, unites our inner world with our outer world and is a portal to our connection with others. Associated with the air element, being aware of our breathing opens us up to the spacious-ness of Self energy in our body. We are aware of the interchange of outside and inside. When consciousness of our breath increases our awareness of the vast space around us, we realize we are all held in a larger container. We draw on that as a resource in our therapeutic work. Just as we receive life-giving oxygen with every breath, when we open to the space around us we may receive guidance from this seeming void.

Awareness of our client's breathing—the rate, the pattern, how it changes over time—gives us information about the inner world of our client, about the state of their autonomic nervous system. Coordinating our breath with our client's helps us get a sense from the inside of what our client is experiencing. We breathe in their inner state and resonate with it, and we send compassion on our outbreath. Simply inviting our client to bring awareness to their breath can be transformative. In addition there are many breathing techniques that can facilitate every step of the IFS process.

Our breathing reminds us of our common dependency on the fragile layer of air that surrounds this planet we share. This awareness unites us with all of life—plants and animals—and dissolves our parts' assumptions about our isolation and differences. We breathe in and our body expands. Our soft palate, our respiratory diaphragm, and our pelvic diaphragm make room to receive the life-giving energies. We breathe out and our body condenses, letting go, feeding the plants. In, out, in, out. Simple awareness makes a shift. Our nervous system is calmed by the rhythmic in and out. The rhythm of our breathing is the counterpoint to the drumbeat of our heart. The heart, nestled snugly in between the lungs, is the first to receive the life-giving air. Both oxygen and *prana* from our lungs nourish the heart, massaging and reassuring the protectors that guard it. With this intimate relationship between the heart and the lungs we gently flow into the relational realms of Radical Resonance.

Just as Somatic Awareness automatically leads us to this practice of Conscious Breathing, Conscious Breathing leads to the next practice, Radical Resonance. Grounding with the earth through Somatic Awareness and opening to the space around us through Conscious Breathing, we establish our vertical alignment. We are in communication and in harmony with energies from above and below. This connection enables us to be a lightning rod for the energies in the therapeutic relationship.

EXERCISES

Bringing Consciousness to Breathing

PURPOSE To become aware of the habitual patterns of your breathing—quality, depth, pace, rhythm, location, body movement—in order to access parts.

INSTRUCTIONS:

1. Appreciate parts that have ideas of "correct" breathing and let them know they can relax during this exercise, whose purpose is to simply bring awareness to your habitual breathing patterns without trying to change them. Let other protector parts know that if, at any point, you begin to feel overwhelmed, you will stop this exercise.

2. Bring your awareness to your breathing in and out. Notice the sensations of taking in the air and letting it out from your nose to your respiratory diaphragm.

3. For several breaths, notice the pace and the rhythm of your breathing.

4. Compare your inhale and your exhale, noticing any differences. Are they equal in length? Does one feel easier or freer than the other?

5. Bring awareness to the places in your body that move as you breathe—top, middle, and lower torso; sides, front, and back. Notice any differences in the movement.

6. Bring awareness to these places in your body that, as you breathe, are not moving as freely. Take some time to study where and how the muscles of your body contribute to restricting fuller breathing.

7. Focus on one aspect of your breathing that you are curious about—the pace, the rhythm, the depth. Explore it for several breaths. You may want to experiment with slightly exaggerating or lessening this aspect.

8. As you are doing this exercise, notice what is happening with your breathing, your awareness, and your emotions.

REFLECTIONS:

1. What did you discover about your habitual breathing pattern?

2. What particular aspect of your breathing interested you?

3. Did bringing your awareness to this aspect lead to any emotions, beliefs, memories, or images? Does this indicate a part?

4. If so, welcome this part and see if it is willing to be known by you. If it seems to be a protector, ask it about its fears, its role, when its behavior started, what it would rather do, what it wants you to know, what it needs from you—anything you are curious about. If it is a vulnerable part, perhaps it is showing you something through your breathing patterns. See if there is anything your parts need right now.

Change Your Breath, Change Your Mind

PURPOSE To bring awareness to the breath to indicate the state of the autonomic nervous system; to learn and practice breathing techniques that regulate emotional states and shift the ANS toward the ventral vagal state.

INSTRUCTIONS:

1. First identify the state of your ANS in this moment, either by noticing your breathing or by being aware of your feelings, or both. If you feel afraid, agitated, or restless, that indicates a sympathetic state. If you are feeling sleepy, dizzy, spacey, collapsed, or disconnected, that indicates a dorsal vagal parasympathetic state.

2. Breathing techniques for addressing sympathetic activation:

   - Square breathing: inhale to the count of four as you imagine drawing the first side of a square, hold your breath for four counts as you draw the second line, exhale for four counts as you draw the third line, and hold your breath as you draw the fourth line. Repeat until you begin to feel calmer.

   - Blowing through a straw: inhale as if you are breathing in through the straw. On the exhale, purse your lips and breathe out long and slowly.

- Ocean breath, or *ujjayi* breath: on the outbreath, contract the muscles of the larynx to add resistance to the exhalation. The sound you make will sound like the waves of the ocean.

- Allow your exhale to gradually be longer than your inhale. Pause at the end of the exhale.

3. Breathing techniques for addressing dorsal vagal activation:

- Breathe deeply into the whole torso, then immediately push the air out, and notice it filling up again. You may sound like a locomotive as the breath gets a bit more rapid and rhythmic. Your belly will draw in toward your spine.

- If you are familiar with pranayama from yoga, you can do the Breath of Fire, which is similar to the previous exercise only faster.

- Stand, arms at sides. Breathe in, lifting your arms, palms facing up, upward toward the ceiling. Breathe out, bringing your arms, palms facing down, back along your sides, drawing your navel toward your spine. Repeat.

- As you exhale, see if there is a sound you want to make. You may first hear it inside—a vowel sound or even a word.

- Let your breathing return to normal. Notice any changes in your breath and your emotional state.

REFLECTIONS:

1. What was your assessment of your ANS state, sympathetic or dorsal vagal?

2. Which breathing techniques did you try? What is the effect?

3. Were any of these exercises particularly helpful for shifting your ANS toward the ventral vagal state of feeling safer and calmer in your body?

4. If so, make an intention to practice the technique, so when you are activated you will be more likely to remember to do it.

Sending Self Energy to a Part through Breath

PURPOSE To use the breath to make space for a part, to bring Self energy to a part, and to assist in an unburdening.

INSTRUCTIONS:

1. Find a comfortable position and bring awareness to several of your breaths. With every inhale, feel the spaciousness in your body. With every exhale, let your awareness go deeper into your inner system.

2. As you deepen, you may find a part that is ready to be known. Invite that part to meet you in your spaciousness you have created for it through your breath.

3. Notice how you feel toward this part. Your breath might give you an embodied clue to how you are feeling. If you are feeling any response other than one that indicates Self energy, that is another part. Locate that part in your body and invite that one into the spaciousness instead of the first one.

4. If you feel some degree of Embodied Self energy toward the part, breathe into where in your body you feel some quality of Self energy, and breathe this energy out to where in your body you feel the part. Do this for several breaths, breathing into Self energy, breathing out Self energy to the part. The part might feel rocked in the rhythm of your breathing.

5. Continue breathing, sending a sound from your Self energy to the part on the exhale. Try different sounds to see which sound touches it. Try "hmmm" and "aaaahh." Notice how the part responds to these sounds.

6. Continue breathing, sending a verbal message along with your breath to the part, such as, "I know," "I am here," or other words that you sense the part needs to hear along with your breath. The part might want a song. It might have a story to tell you.

7. If you sense the part is ready to let go of what it is carrying—fear, shame, the belief that it is alone, pain, tension—you can invite the part to use the outbreath to give this burden to the air, to the infinite space.

8. Take some more breaths to come to a completion with this part.

REFLECTIONS (journal or share)

1. What part showed up in the space you created?

2. If it was difficult to feel some quality of Self energy toward the part, what part was it that had some fear or concern? Was it helped by your breath?

3. What was your part's experience as you breathed your Self energy to it?

4. Was it able to let go of a burden?

4

Radical Resonance:
Potentiating Relational Realms

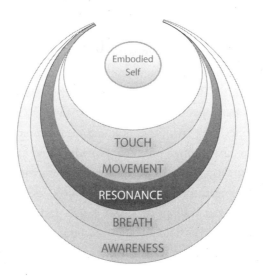

ROOTED IN THE EARTHY foundation of Somatic Awareness and enlivened by the air of Conscious Breathing bridging our inner and outer worlds, the practice of Radical Resonance takes us beyond the vertical plane to explore the rich complexity of the horizontal field. Aligned with the earth and the sky, nourished and strengthened by the many energies from above and below, our vertical alignment buttresses us as we venture into this territory brimming with relationship.

To help with the transition from the vertical to the horizontal planes of relationship, some of my clients like to begin the session with a short walking meditation. My client and I stand side by side. We connect with the ground by jiggling our body, wiggling our toes, and feeling our bones. We connect with the sky and the space around us by noticing our breathing, reaching up with our arms over our head. We begin to walk and breathe together in a particular way, consciously connecting with the earth on the first step, and with the sky on the second step, occasionally pausing to gather up the energies of earth and sky into our heart. This pause reinforces the balance of living—returning to the vertical to rest and reboot and then venturing again into the horizontal to the vulnerable territory of inner and outer relationships.

It can get messy as we step out into the world of relationship. Our internal systems can be complex, and interpersonal systems offer more complexity and more opportunity. The relational dance is risky and delicate. Our parts bump into others' parts, like stones tossed by the waves. We bump into each other and, like stones, we either break or knock off the rough points. Awareness of this vertical line through our body provides a keel as we navigate the winding and often choppy waters of relationship. Awareness of the vertical line of energy running through our body also affects our posture. We can breathe better. Our heart is supported. Our organs don't feel squashed. Our neck doesn't have to strain to hold up our seven-pound cranium. Connecting with stability and support from the earth and wisdom from the infinite space above us, we dare to enter this more complex and often uncertain realm of relationship.

The first recorded usage of the word "relationship" was in the 1700s, and two hundred years later it was referring specifically to romantic or sexual relationships. In the last several decades this word has taken on a much more general definition. In Somatic IFS we consider the healing power of resonance specifically in regard to the relationship between the Embodied Self (of either therapist or client) and the parts of the internal system, although we recognize that resonance can be transformative in any intimate relationship.

We are in relationship from the moment of conception. Our earliest experiences become the template of our later relational behaviors. These implicit stories are recorded subcortically, in our brain and body, and are played out in our parts' behaviors. The "known but not remembered" early attachment experiences are expressed in posture, gesture, muscular contractions, breathing patterns, dissociation, and sexual energy. Through these raw, elegant, primitive poetics, parts' early relational wounds resonate in the Embodied Self of client and therapist.

What Is Resonance?

"Resonance" is a term widely used in the fields of acoustics, physics, chemistry, and electricity to refer to the interaction of vibrating systems. Every object has a natural frequency, and resonance describes the phenomenon happening when music being played in a room causes a vase in the room to vibrate. When the objects vibrate at a comparable frequency, the objects oscillate with a greater amplitude. Resonance is the codependent dynamic interaction of two coupled systems. The resonant interaction in Somatic IFS includes both amplifying and syncing with the vibrations of parts and Self co-created within the dyadic system and within larger systems.

As a clarinet player getting in tune with another instrument, I could hear the oscillating vibrations move into coherence as we got in tune. If my note was slightly higher or lower than another's, I heard a beating sound within the pitch, kind of like "wah-wah-wah." As I got more in tune, the beats became slower and slower until the sound waves were in sync and there was no detectable beat. The satisfaction of becoming more "in tune" in order to make music is similar to how it feels to attune to the somatic soundtrack of my clients' early relational traumas that accompany their verbal stories and join in a somatic duet as our energies come into a greater coherence.

Scientists have measured the electromagnetic frequency of Earth's vibration and tell us that in addition to objects, all living things have particular vibratory frequencies that can be measured, including all the structures of the human body. The seemingly solid human body, according to Einstein, is energy whose vibration is low enough that we can perceive it. It turns out that the resonant frequency of the planet matches that of our cells, and of human consciousness during the alpha brain wave state (our quiet or meditative times). There is evidence that our vibrations speed up when we are on our electronic devices, and scientists tell us the natural pulse of Earth, called Schumann's resonance, is also speeding up. It seems likely that, if measured, our various parts would have different frequencies and the wavelength of Self energy would be more in sync with the pulse of the planet.

Resonance in Somatic IFS views a relationship as the flow of energy and information between parts and Self. Intimate relationships, including the therapeutic relationship, reveal the body-based attachment experiences. The energy and information of these experiences are transmitted as vibrational frequencies via bodies and right-brain structures. These psychobiological roots of our relational experiences from conception through infancy are brought to awareness through somatic practices. The resonant body is the vehicle for the psychobiological attunement of Self energy necessary to receive the early stories and to rewire habitual patterns of relating. Just as one instrument sounding a perfect C pitch can bring into coherence an instrument playing slightly off-key, an individual in Self energy resonating with the frequency of the parts can bring those frequencies into coherence with the frequency of Self energy.

A client enters therapy with all their protectors on high alert, assuming they will be rejected, humiliated, or abandoned if they disclose any sign of vulnerability. Their parts are gathering information about the level of safety and acceptance in the relationship. Much of the energy and information that signals a safe, resonant relationship is transmitted nonverbally, as right-brain-to-right-brain communication, often below the level of awareness. The therapist, open to receiving the energetic vibrations of the client's parts, can amplify and bring into coherence those vibrations that might have been just dimly felt. The client's inner system may at first—and most likely at many times throughout the therapy process—rely on the therapist to be the vehicle of resonance until the parts can trust the Self of the client to be the secure attachment figure for their wounded parts.

The implicit stories of the parts' neuronally based and embodied relational patterns floating in the intersubjective, often turbulent waters of the therapeutic relationship compel a response that may require therapists to descend into the mysteries of their own bodymind. The clarity of Self energy prevents floundering in an empathic puddle of emotions. Rather than being an observer or even an experienced guide, the therapist reverberates with the tremors of abuse, neglect, betrayal, and abandonment. The parts' tacit stories feel fathomed. Their burdened beliefs about rejection and isolation dissolve in the emotional, right-brain watery relational realm.

The client's own Embodied Self energy emerges as the secure attachment figure for the client's young parts. The vibrations of Embodied Self energy in both therapist and client are amplified. The resulting energies are more than an additive process, greater than transmission or contagion. The dynamic interplay co-created within the relational field multiplies the Embodied Self energy exponentially.

Why *Radical* Resonance?

The adjective "radical" that describes this practice, in addition to being conveniently alliterative, accentuates the deeply rooted quality of a resonant relationship. When in relationship our senses and our hearts are open and every cell seems alive, the experience is as radical as it gets. "Radical" comes from the Latin *radicalis,* which means "having roots." The state of resonance is not a shallow experience of connection. It is not gliding on the surface and offering therapeutic platitudes. It is only when we are connected through our roots—as with plants that intertwine roots or grow from the same root stock—that we can provide the kind of radical connection that makes a deep trust possible.

Peter Wohlleben in his book *The Hidden Life of Trees* writes of electrical impulses that pass through the roots of trees by means of fungi in the soil.[1] It seems that isolated trees and trees planted for agricultural reasons have lost these abilities. At the root, at the most fundamental level, living beings thirst for resonance with other living beings. Some of our clients, like the isolated or farmed tree, have lost their ability to establish a safe, rooted connection with a fellow human being. Protective parts, determined that the client never again suffer injuries at the hands of other people, have numbed and distorted their sensory capacity to read the signals of safety. Unlike trees, though, parts that have blocked the innate capacity to differentiate between danger and safety in relationships can be healed. The repair begins with the therapist, flexibly and fluidly synchronizing with the client's state and transmitting Embodied Self energy. It begins with the therapist trusting that this energy is powerfully transformative.

With this practice we are delving into the mysterious domain of what is thought to be beyond our ability to perceive or measure—at least if we look only through a Newtonian lens. Viewing through this lens we are likely to dismiss the exchange of energy between client and therapist as being "woo woo." Quantum physics has revealed that atoms are made out of invisible energy, not tangible matter, and that these laws apply at every level of the universe. Matter can be understood as both a solid particle and as a wave. Matter and energy are interdependent and interconnected. It turns out that, at the root, we are far more connected than we can perceive or even imagine.

The reality of a quantum universe reunites the Cartesian separation of mind and matter that has dominated Western thought and practices. Quantum physics reunites us with our ancient roots, revealing that matter and energy are completely entangled, leading to a worldview not unlike that of our most ancient ancestors and some still surviving indigenous cultures who believe that rocks, water, air, and animals—including humans—are all equally imbued with spirit, with invisible energy. Today some cultures, such as Australian aborigines and Amazonian shamans, still utilize their energy-sensing capacities, and so they have not atrophied as have most of ours in developed civilizations. Thousands of years before Western scientists discovered the laws of quantum physics, Eastern healing practices measured and treated the energy imbalances that contribute to physical, emotional, and spiritual diseases. If most of the energy exchange in our therapy offices is below the level of our awareness, we can begin by being aware that we are not aware of it. With intention and receptivity, our ability to sense energy transmissions can develop.

Today I was meditating with my sangha of about a dozen people. I was sitting next to a woman who had recently been diagnosed with breast cancer. Her head was covered because her hair was beginning to fall out from the chemotherapy. As my mind and body began to settle, I sensed a big ball of warm energy rising up from my belly to my head, and tears began to flow down my face and my nose began to run. I checked with my parts to see if any of them were sad, and it was clear the sadness was not coming from my inner system. I also felt some vague sensations on the right side of my body. I noticed this woman sitting at my right, sniffling, looking for a tissue, and struggling to sit quietly. She shifted on her pillow and frequently looked at her watch. When it was time for walking meditation I went with her into another room and sat with her. After a few tears and a little talk, her body, reacting to the strong chemicals flooding it, shifted into a state where she could rejoin the group. She shared with me that her illness is compelling her to write a book she has had in mind for over a decade. Her presence impacted our entire sangha, probably in ways beyond our level of awareness. I noticed our group seemed even more openhearted and cohesive.

Charles was participating in an exercise in a Somatic IFS retreat practicing Radical Resonance. His partner was sharing about his fear of making mistakes, and Charles began to have a hard time breathing. He asked for my help, and together we found a part that had the same fear as his partner of making mistakes. Charles's part was making such an extreme effort to resonate perfectly that it was causing a crushing pressure in his chest. His part had been pressured by his immigrant parents to succeed. He imagined placing his hand on the young part's back behind his heart and spoke reassuringly to the boy. He unburdened the perfectionism and efforting in both this part and in his parents. His breathing returned to normal, his heart felt open. His partner in the exercise, rather than feeling abandoned while Charles worked with his part, told him his own efforting part unburdened along with him, and he felt more relaxed, too.

Perhaps resonance takes us to where the ideas of therapist and client, self and other begin to dissolve, expanding beyond interpersonal, intrapersonal, and transpersonal healing to establish a more harmonious relationship with other human beings, with all living beings, with the planet, even with the universe. Perhaps restoring our ability to resonate could heal our narcissistic parts' view that we have the right to dominate other people, animals, Earth. Maybe it could result in more social and economic equality. Instead of continuing our practice of controlling Earth's resources for our own gain, we could avoid the sixth mass extinction where over a million species will disappear from the planet. Perhaps this dream begins with the courage to radically resonate with another's pain.

Radical Resonance Is Associated with the Water Element

The waves of Lake Michigan make a low chuckle as they innocently lap the rocks on the shore near my home. The gentle sound of the moving water belies the power of the water to turn the rocks into grains of sand that will be blown into a dune by the wind. Just by moving freely and continuously, water patiently, powerfully, and thoroughly washes over any obstacle, clearing away and carrying away the residue, eventually flushing it downstream to the ocean. Drop by drop it wears away stone. Water teaches us about relationships and the process of change. Resonating with pain in a fully embodied way eventually dissolves the hard places of hurt. Just as water wears away rock and ocean currents actually reshape the earth's solid forms, the practice of Radical Resonance can reshape the neural firing patterns in the brain and revise other chemical and energetic patterns in the body.

Our lives began with water. Life on our planet began when molecules in a primordial soup or a vent deep in the ocean made the shift to a living cell. Each of us begins life as a water creature. The fertilized egg floats in the amniotic sea, and as it develops there is a state where the human embryo resembles the fish embryo, with slits and gill arches. Our cells communicate with each other and re-create themselves as they move through their watery world. The fluids inside the cell exchange substances within the interstitial fluids that bathe every cell. The fluid movement resembles the jellyfish's pulsating movement. The cells of the embryo, having developed through the expanding and condensing of cellular fluids, grow our head, tail, and four limbs. The patterns of a water creature remain even though we build on these patterns to be able to walk on land. As Emilie Conrad writes, "The human body has been spiraled from the vortical tendency of living water, an extension of the primordial ocean, appearing separate but maintaining constant resonance. We are in perpetual rapport with all fluid systems *everywhere in the universe,* functioning as an undivided whole."[2]

The potential of a Self-led relationship is similar to the qualities of water. Water slakes our thirst. Water dissolves, cleanses, and purifies. Water softens the hard, parched earth and restores life to what had become withered. Water is transformational. Water itself changes from liquid to solid to vapor. Whatever forms water takes—mist, raindrop, pond, river, lake— eventually all find their way to the ocean and merge into one.

Water is considered the element of the unconscious and associated with intuition, emotion, empathy, and psychic energy. Like the unconscious, the surface of a deep lake may be calm or riffled by the wind. The reflected light may obscure the hidden depths. Our emotions, like water, want to flow. Dammed by fears or shame they stagnate. When they break free, waves of raging waters may flood the system and crash against the shore. When the emotions and energies find a safe channel they gently flow downward toward a harbor of stillness and peace.

In aikido I learned a simple exercise where I hold my arm outstretched as I visualize my energy flowing from my core out through my fingertips like water through a fire hose. The exercise demonstrated that this visualization made my arm far stronger than when I attempted to tighten against the force of a downward push. Applying this aikido principle to the therapeutic relationship, we connect with our core—the core of our body and the central reason we are together. We notice parts' reactions to our clients' resistances or pushing. We connect with our fluid nature and the deeper waters that nourish our entwined roots. The relational waters flow, clearing away any sluggish pools and frozen or parched places within us, and our resonance can offer this fluidity to soften the client's tightly bound protectors.

Water metaphors abound as we consider the relational process of therapy. Sitting with our client at the beginning of a session it is as if we sit by a dark lake and wonder about the temperature, the consistency of the lake bottom, the life within. Our interactions may be like a pebble thrown into still waters. The pebble sinks out of sight and the ripples form ever-widening circles. The pebble may ripple within the depths of our psyche as well, stirring up unresolved fear, longing, despair.

The client's inner sea begins to stir and something bubbles up from the dark waters. Some raw emotion—sadness, anger, or anxiety—rises to the surface. We listen to our client's speech—the tone, pace, amplitude, tempo, rhythm, prosody—as well as facial expressions, breath, posture, eye gaze, and gestures for clues to what is lurking under the surface of the words. Their parts' emotions may begin to flood their systems. Our client senses us journeying with them in their rough seas. We are also tossed about, and our own undigested emotions in the depths of our bodymind may be stirred. We keep our head above water by connecting with the tidal rhythms of breath and heartbeat and the longer rhythms of expansion and contraction. Our inner sea calms, and that calm presence is transmitted through our eye gaze, our breath, our posture, our voice tone as well as words. Our Embodied Self energy can act as anchor, buoy, or lighthouse as our client's inner world is revealed and witnessed, and the burdens are dissolved in the relational waters.

Resonance in History and in Contemporary Practice

As with Conscious Breathing, the roots of the practice of resonance reach deep both in spirituality and in science. In the thirteenth century, the poet and mystic Mevlana Jelaluddin Rumi invited us to let go of ideas of right-doing and wrong-doing so we could lie down in the grass of a non-dual, resonant relational field. In the history of psychotherapy, there are many references to the state of resonance with various labels. Wilhelm Reich used the terms "vegetative identification" and "organic transference" to refer to the physiological interpersonal regulation that results from the nonconscious interaction between therapist and client.[3] Carl Jung's theory of "collective unconscious" describes a mode of shared informational patterns.[4] Resting on the shoulders of Reich and Jung, Stanley Keleman, a leader in body psychotherapy, first used the term "somatic resonance" for the biological rapport between two people.[5]

Many contemporaries recognize the centrality of resonance in healing relationships. Radical Resonance, as it involves affective and psychobiological processes, is no longer restricted to the realm of the touchy-feely, New Age, marginally respected therapists. Contemporary psychoanalysts refer to "relational unconscious" for the nonverbal communication between the unconscious minds of therapist and client. Recent intensive interdisciplinary research is transforming psychotherapy from the behavioral and cognitive focus to include the psychobiological processes as they relate to the therapeutic relationship.

The explosion of discoveries in neuroscience and attachment theory over the last thirty years has expanded and validated our understanding of this phenomenon. Neuroscientists are discovering how and where in the brain this seemingly mysterious unconscious communication happens. They have taught us about the social engagement system, the role of the amygdala, insula, and prefrontal cortex, the mirror neurons and the bonding hormones, and the resonance circuits. We understand how this information confirms the neural plasticity of the brain. Realizing the potential for psychobiological attunement to rewire brains damaged by trauma and faulty attachment, therapists are committed to applying this wellspring of information to their clients. The practice of Radical Resonance is the key to this healing.

Neuropsychologist Allan Schore concisely describes the phenomenon of resonance as "implicit, nonverbal, affect-laden right-brain communication."[6] His research of mothers and children and therapists and their patients supports the idea that brains can be reorganized and regulated in both kinds of relationships. Both mothers and therapists can serve as "interactive psychobiological regulators." A major tenet of his work is that in relationship, while the left brain communicates via conscious language, the right brain is communicating its unconscious states nonverbally to receptive right brains with bodily based emotional empathy.

Other researchers have used various adjectives to modify "resonance." Laurie Carr uses the term "empathic resonance."[7] Using functional MRI to map brain activity during observation and imitation of emotional facial expressions, researchers found that our empathic resonance is grounded in the emotions associated with body movement. Biologist Rupert Sheldrake extends the concept of resonance beyond the interpersonal to the transpersonal.[8] He speaks of "morphic resonance" as a cumulative memory of similar systems through cultures and time. He hypothesizes that all biological systems, from molecules to bodies to societies and even entire galaxies, are shaped by morphic fields. These fields have a resonance that reverberates across generations with an inherent memory that shapes and organizes living systems. Bonnie Bainbridge Cohen of Body-Mind Centering uses the term "cellular resonance" to describe the reciprocal relationship between the cells of the body, between humans, between other life forms, and even with the universe.[9]

Psychiatrist and pioneer brain researcher Daniel Siegel has written extensively about the interpersonal dance between the biological and psychological systems of two beings in a significant relationship. In *The Mindful Therapist* Siegel describes resonance as the mutually transformative aspect of intimate relationships. His theory of "interpersonal neurobiology" defines a relationship as the sharing of the flow of energy and information (energy with meaning and symbolism). The body, including the brain, is the mechanism of that flow, and the mind is the self-organizing embodied and relational process that regulates this flow of energy and information located within an individual and between individuals in relationship. This interaction stimulates the activity and growth of fibers in the brain to repair relational wounds and leads to greater brain integration. When we are willing to be impacted in a relationship, we impact others. He tells us that in some cases "shifts in EEG and heart rate variability co-occur. The functions of our autonomic nervous system . . . become aligned and we resonate with each other . . . Our job is not to be the one who knows everything, but the one who is present, attuned, and open for what is."[10]

It seems we are not the separate autonomous individuals our parts imagine. It is not just the client's brain that is transformed but the therapist's as well. Siegel tells us, "Resonance reveals the deep reality that we are a part of a larger whole . . . that we are created by the ongoing dance within, between and among us."[11] The "dance" can be an intrapersonal one as we tune in to and express our body's rhythm. We can take it to the interpersonal level as we find another person on the dance floor and allow our dance to be impacted by another's rhythm. And the relational dance can take us to the edge of the transpersonal. When we each allow ourselves to be impacted by the internal state of our partner, the dance that we co-create is one of coherence and harmony. We may find that we are dancing "the ongoing dance within, between and among us." When we attune, the circuitry of our nervous system is such that "we come to create resonance in which our observing self takes on some of the features of that which we are observing."[12]

Siegel points to the process by which a healing relationship can occur. He describes the process with an acronym: ironically, PART. P stands for presence, or mindful awareness and a state of receptivity to what is emerging in the relational field. Presence has been shown to raise the enzyme levels to repair and maintain the ends of chromosomes to keep cells healthy. The A is for attunement—the focusing of attention on the internal experience of another person as well as ourselves. R is for resonating, which Siegel describes as including both linkage and differentiation—not becoming the person, but feeling their feelings so that it changes you and allows the other person to "feel felt." Trust, which can be measured physiologically, emerges in a relationship of presence, attunement, and resonance, represented by the letter T.

Jack Kornfield, one of the key teachers to introduce Buddhist mindfulness practice to the West and who brilliantly incorporates Eastern philosophy with Western psychology, describes limbic resonance: "If a person filled with panic or hatred walks into a room, we feel it immediately, and unless we are very mindful, that person's negative state will begin to overtake our own. When a joyfully expressive person walks into a room, we can feel that state as well."[13] Kornfield and Siegel have occasionally joined their Buddhist psychology and neuroscience-informed mindsight to share their explorations of brain, mind, and spirit and to teach practices that help others find a resilient and vibrant way to be in our challenging world.

Before I became familiar with Siegel's work, the book that awakened me to the reciprocal nature of resonance and the resultant revision of our brain was *A General Theory of Love*. The mysteries of love and connection are explored by three psychiatrists drawing from brain research—particularly the limbic structures of the brain. They use the term "limbic resonance," which they describe as "a symphony of mutual exchange and internal adaptation whereby two mammals become attuned to each other's inner states."[14] This innate capacity, they tell us, is the basis of social connection and especially of our healing, loving relationships. "Limbic states can leap between minds . . . the limbic activity of those around us draws our emotions into almost immediate congruence."[15] They cite research that suggests limbic resonance actually revises damaged subcortical structures in caregiver and infant, and in therapist and client.

Systems of the Body
Associated with Radical Resonance

Fluids

Like our planet, the human body is about two-thirds water. Over half the body's fluids are within the cells, and another quarter surrounds the cells. This interstitial fluid contains sugars, salts, hormones, amino acids, fatty acids, neurotransmitters, cellular waste products. The fluid inside the cell is viscous, containing nutrients and structures that carry out the essential work of the cell. We access the qualities of fluidity and responsivity by bringing awareness to the body's fluids and the organs associated with these fluids. Our blood plasma, lymph, interstitial fluid, cranial sacral fluid, and synovial fluid all are continuously circulating and contributing to homeostasis.

Communication and transformation of inner and outer environments happens in our body fluids. These fluids can become blocked. Our parts' burdens can be held in the fluids of the body. Linda Hartley of Body-Mind Centering makes a connection between the blocked or distorted flow of these fluids and a related blockage in the mind from repressed or unexpressed emotions. She has found that awareness of the natural flow of the fluids helps repattern the flow and release "stagnating" emotions.

What we observe and experience is that repressed or unexpressed emotional experiences can be held within the fluids of the body; it may be that the body fluids attract the charge of emotional energy in a way similar to that of water acting as a conductor for electrical energy. These held emotions can stagnate in the same way as a river does when blocked, until awareness of the natural flow is reawakened there; through this awareness the fluids themselves can be repatterned.[16]

Studying with another practitioner of Body-Mind Centering, Lisa Clark, I have discovered that becoming more familiar with my fluid nature has increased my resonant capacity. When guided to drop into "body time" so as to tune in to these various fluids, I began to experience that each fluid has its own quality, its own rhythm. The rhythm of the blood feels like the waves of the ocean; the arterial flow is like a wave rushing toward the shore, while the venous flow is like the wave pulling away from the sand to gather strength; each offers a different aspect of relational resonance. I learned that the lymph arises from the plasma of the arterial blood. Like the blood, it flows from periphery to core. Unlike the blood, it relies on movement for its flow. Moving while focusing on my lymph system, I feel a sense of clarity in relationship. I learned that our blood, lymph, cerebral spinal fluid, and synovial fluid all arise out of the interstitial fluid surrounding our cells. Clark teaches that the rhythmic movement of fluids into and out of the cell is the foundation of later development—of our movement patterns and the related emotions, beliefs, and behaviors.

From my experience as a cranial sacral therapist I have been familiar with the qualities of cerebral spinal fluid. As this cranial sacral fluid (CSF) is produced and absorbed in structures in the brain, there are subtle rhythmic waves of movement throughout the body. Attending to the slow pulsation is deeply relaxing for both myself and my client, and together we enter into an egoless, oceanic state. Bainbridge Cohen says that through the CSF we contact the "central core of unbounded self."[17] This fluid has taught me about resonant relationships. I need to first become grounded before I make contact. My touch as a cranial sacral practitioner is as light as a feather—much different from digging into my client's fascial restrictions. Tension anywhere in my body interferes with my ability to sense the subtle rhythmic waves. As the fluid moves the membranes and bones of the body, I pay attention to the tides and the waves rather than assessing, judging, and correcting any dysfunction. My hands gently follow the abnormal rhythm, the asymmetry, the sluggish flow, witnessing it, supporting it, possibly exaggerating it. In response to this touch, the rhythm of the CSF system eventually comes to a stop. This pause in the habitual behavior, like a self-initiated time-out, is referred to as a "still point." During this pause, the system reorganizes in a more optimal pattern, with a more robust, even, and symmetrical movement. Many clients free emotional burdens during this process. I have never lost the thrill of experiencing how the dysfunctional system quite organically and paradoxically resets itself into a preferred pattern. From countless experiences I learned to trust that mindful attention supports the inherent self-correcting of the system.

Our Magical Cell "Mem-Brain"

The cell communicates with other cells through its external environment. Each cell has an astonishing ability to sense the internal and external environment and to make appropriate behavior changes. Each cell membrane demonstrates the creativity and intelligence to know what to let in and receive and what to let go of. Its job is protection. It is responsive to its environment and is influenced by and influences other cells. Cells communicate with each other via the interstitial fluid through the cell membrane. The relationship between the cell and its external environment is a microcosm of an interpersonal relationship.

Cellular biologist Bruce Lipton performed breakthrough studies on the cellular membrane that integrate the principles of quantum physics with our understanding of cellular biology. In *The Biology of Belief* Lipton describes the action of the cell membrane at the molecular level where receptor and effector proteins function as the cell's intelligence. Receptor proteins receive information about the environment—both internal and external to the cell. They read vibrational energy fields and vibrate like tuning forks. The effector proteins generate cellular behavior. To study the membrane's perception switches that shift the cell's behavior, Lipton experimented with cells that line the blood vessels; he found that even these single cells reach out for nourishment and recoil from noxious or toxic substances. The semipermeable membrane chooses what molecules to let in and what to keep out, what to hold on to and what to let go of. In this way, life and growth occur.[18]

Each individual's bodymind has a more complex version of a semipermeable membrane with capacities to receive and to effect action in response to what is received. The brain takes on the job of the cell membrane: receiving information from the internal and external environments, regulating and moderating the internal system. The limbic system receives information from cells throughout the body and generates emotions through the release of signals by the nervous system. Yet the individual cell retains its intelligence. Candace Pert, as described in her book *Molecules of Emotion,* discovered that the neural receptors in the brain are present in most of the body's cells, establishing that the "mind" does not exist in the head but in the entire body.[19] Our parts' beliefs, conscious as well as unconscious, are held in our cells and affect every cell of our body. With our brain and the receptor proteins of our "mem-brain" we perceive and interpret signals of safety or lack of it. We make choices about what to let in and what to keep out, what to retain and what no longer is needed.

Like our cells, we are semipermeable to each other's emotional states. We observe each other's nonverbal signals and make meaning of that data, but we also vibrate, often below our conscious awareness, with energy fields. In a process similar to osmosis, we are influenced by each other's emotions or Self energy. We all experience the permeability of moods, attitudes, and emotional fields. We also have filters and boundaries. Some emotions may bead up like rain droplets on a window or may slide off like fried eggs on a Teflon pan. We may take in certain protective attitudes of criticism or defensiveness just deeply enough to be able to get a whiff of the underlying vulnerability. Emotions, like smells, flow into our inner systems. We detect discomfort or awkwardness that may indicate our client's semipermeable boundaries are locking in feelings to avoid shame or judgment. We sense into the block as well as the longing to reveal the depths of despair or rage. Our thirst for connection in emotional health is as essential as water in our physical health. Perhaps bringing awareness to this magical and intelligent structure around every one of our trillions of cells can assist us in our resonant relationships.

The Limbic Brain

Lizards lack the limbic brain. They lay their eggs in the sand and slither away. Mammals have this brain. Because of this brain they cuddle and croon to their young. The limbic brain, nestled between the reptilian brain and the neocortex, is an evolutionary development that allows us greater social and emotional intelligence. As described earlier in this chapter, the limbic brain is the repository of emotions where our early relational patterns are encoded entirely in implicit memory. It is also where the neural deficits can be modified by new experiences. Healthy, Self-led interactions can harness this neural plasticity to rewire neurons in more optimal ways. New neural circuits and pathways can be created by interactions with an attuned, accepting therapist.

Neuroscientists have identified some structures, including mirror neurons, involved in Radical Resonance. Their research contends that we are hardwired to make somatic shifts in relation to another person. When we attune to our client's behavior, their gestures, tone of voice, and facial expressions, mirror neurons fire in our brain. This information travels quickly from the cortex through the insula and through the limbic regions to the neurons of interoception. This process ties into Somatic Awareness, helping us know what we are feeling in our body. Our mirror neurons allow for subcortical resonance, giving us a sense—from the inside out—of what our clients are feeling. Our limbic structures attribute an emotional meaning to our body sensations, and the information travels on to the middle prefrontal cortex, which is involved with empathy and resonance, qualities that are most effectively communicated to our clients nonverbally. The mirror neuron system illuminates the profoundly social nature of the brain.

The Heart

Although the brain is involved in Radical Resonance, the heart is by far the strongest resonating organ. Heart cells are the first cells to form in the embryo, and the body grows and is organized in the heart field. The heart is far more than a pump for our blood. Since the dawn of civilization, the heart has been considered to be the center of our feelings and our ability to love. Research from the HeartMath Institute shows that the heart is surrounded by a large, powerful field, about ten feet in diameter, and that it produces the strongest magnetic and electrical impulses in the body, five thousand times more powerful than the electromagnetic field created by the brain.

It is possible that the heart has declarative memory. In 1998 psycho-neuroimmunologist Paul Pearsall[20] conducted research with heart transplant recipients, including an eight-year-old recipient whose donor had been murdered; the child remembered all the details of the murder, even being able to identify the murderer. From his research Pearsall concludes the cells of the heart have memory. Pearsall further claims that the whole body is an info-energetic intelligence field and that it is the heart rather than the brain that primarily directs the body's systems.

Although there are skeptics who question body memory and cellular memory, I rely foremost on my direct experience to speak of the heart's relevance to Radical Resonance. I cannot feel sensations in my limbic brain structures to verify experientially what researchers have found, but I can feel sensations in and around my heart. In relationship I find sensations of either warmth and openness or a wall, a block, a blankness. My students, supervisees, and clients also find both sensations, which indicate parts or Self in their hearts. Our parts, not recognizing the power and resiliency of this center of relationality, fear its vulnerability. Fearing the pain of old wounds of broken-heartedness when we felt abandoned and mistreated, our parts cover our heart with layers of protection, insulating it against our own and the world's pain. With less access to our heart, we overdevelop the ability to listen with our ears and brain. We focus on the content in order to get the facts straight and remember them. Just as our brain is hardwired to resonate and has the ability to revise a damaged limbic system, one open heart can transmit healing energy to another heart. In a healing relationship, we unburden these parts and uncover our heart's natural ability to resonate. According to Daniel Siegel, relationship is the sharing of the flow of energy and information, and this flow flows from one heart to another.

None of these body systems operate independently of the others. In fact, the heart and the brain, which in the embryo are almost touching each other, have a strong communication system throughout our life. James Doty, a Stanford neurosurgeon and director of the Center for Compassion and Altruism Research and Education, is on the cutting edge of our understanding how the brain and heart talk to each other.[21] He speaks of the two-way street of neural enervation flowing between the brain stem and heart, which can reshape our fight and flight responses. His particular hope is that what he refers to as our "baggage of evolution" of tribal conflict may be reshaped by the resonant communication between heart and brain. His research on what compassion means in the body and in action has implications not only for our individual lives but for our society.

The Body as Consultant

As therapists we know the importance of boundaries and differentiation. We have believed it is important to discern whether a body symptom is ours or our client's. Radical Resonance implies that body sensations emerge within the intersubjective field of the therapeutic relationship. Our parts may fear the intimacy of this radical connection. Our own relational traumas may be triggered. It may be our fears rather than a client's "resistance" that interfere with the therapeutic relationship, creating somatic dissonance rather than resonance. It is essential for us as therapists and practitioners to know the triggers that block our resonance, so we can restore our body's inherent ability to receive and to reverberate with the energies and information floating in the relational bio-field. Whose symptom it is matters less than what we do with it.

In the early days of teaching IFS, I had stomachaches that disappeared as soon as I was no longer in front of the group. I assumed it was nerves, but when I checked inside I found a part that was using this body symptom to let me know that there was something lurking in the depths of the group that needed my attention. Of course I knew that every group, until there is enough safety, is rife with hidden fears, insecurities, competitions, and polarizations, and I didn't need a stomachache—sometimes so intense it interfered with my ability to be present—to remind me. I separated from parts that wanted the pain to go away. I thanked the part for its ability to resonate with the group's energies and let it know I got the message. I told the part I could listen better if it would lower the signal. The discomfort soon resolved as I attended to my body's subtle messages and learned to flow with the stream of the group's hopes and fears.

With individual clients we don't automatically assume that physical symptoms arising are necessarily "ours," but we consider they may be offering information about the client and the relationship. Nausea, headache, agitation, restriction, tension, and dissociation may be synchronous body states that emerge within the resonant field of the therapeutic relationship. Boredom may be a sign that the process is not on track. Frustration may indicate that the client's anger is being exiled. Sleepiness may indicate the client is moving toward dissociation. The therapy relationship may mirror the client's other intimate relationships. These symptoms may be giving us important information about our client's inner worlds, and we welcome them as valuable consultants and invite them to share their information.

Receptivity and Revision

So many words concerning a resonant relationship also start with the letter R, like receptivity and revision. There's also reciprocity, rapport . . . and reactivity and ruptures. And, hopefully, repair. Many of these words also have the "re" root, meaning "again and again" or "turning back toward something." In relationship we return to our roots of perception, to interoception, to find an openness to receive the signals. Receptivity allows for resonance, and resonance allows for what neuroscientists have termed "revision." We have learned from their research that the somatic contagion occurring in a resonant relationship involves many body systems. The social engagement system of the autonomic nervous system, the fight-or-flight response of the amygdala, mirror neurons, bonding hormones, the social-emotional bias of the right hemisphere and the prefrontal cortex—all play a role in therapeutic change.

Receptivity

Radical Resonance depends on the therapist's ability to be receptive to the client's emotional energies. We are inherently receptive, but this capacity can be disrupted by our parts that believe this is a risky endeavor. Being open is what got them in trouble, they will say; it's much safer to close off. Parts may fear being pulled into an emotional vortex and becoming flooded by pain and so erect a barrier. It can be a hard sell for our parts to step back enough for us to receive our client's pain—energetically, emotionally, and physically. Similar to a resonating object that is touched, our receptivity to our client's energies can be blocked or disrupted by parts. Instead of resonance, we experience somatic dissonance. The receptive capacity may be either suppressed, such as when we feel bored, numb, or tired, or heightened, such as when we feel distracted, agitated, or anxious.

When I am consulting with other therapists, I consider how to help regulate their receptivity, and I may suggest the therapist find a different place in their body to receive the vibrational energy of their clients, where it can be modulated for most effective receptivity. For example, Jackie found shifting her open receptivity to the back of her body to help her with a client.

Jackie is an exceptionally empathic and sensitive therapist. I am in awe of her ability to somatically receive so much energy and information from her client. Jackie describes her session with a client, and she conveys to me a vivid sense of her client's parts—the one that had been abandoned when her father left the family, her manager's desperation to be able to function better in her life, her vulnerable parts desperately looking to Jackie for rescue, and her firefighter part that could cut her off as easily as a hot knife through butter. I can even feel some resonance with her client in my own body, thirdhand.

Jackie is so open to sensing her client's unarticulated emotions and beliefs that she herself is quivering with her own raw emotions. She recognizes some personal parallels with her client's issues. She is blended with parts that are afraid of being judged and abandoned by her client. Jackie feels deeply attached to her client and is open to the emotional energies reverberating between them, but the vibrations are so strong she loses the ballast of Self energy. She feels she has lost her "therapist eyes." As I consider how to help Jackie, I tune in to my own body, wondering what allows me to have these therapist eyes. Simply because I am not sitting with Jackie's client, I feel an empathic connection with her client but not strong enough to overtake my Self energy.

Wondering how I can help Jackie, I feel my awareness being drawn to the back of my body. When I connect to others from the front of my body I seem to relate with more vulnerability and softness. The back of my body offers a more boundaried experience of relating. I suggest to Jackie that she tune in to the back of her body. She touches along her body from the top of her head, through her ears, down her shoulders, along the sides of her torso and legs. From this awareness of the frontal plane separating her front and back body, she appreciates her front body for being so open, so viscerally receptive to her clients' emotional lives. She begins to experiment with how it might be to walk from, and to perceive from, her back body. Because all our habits are deeply rooted, she first practices relating through her back body and then begins to apply it in the therapist chair.

Our body is naturally receptive and knows how to regulate. Our cell membranes know how to be selective in what they take in and what they hold on to. Perhaps we can trust in this wisdom to absorb just enough emotional energy to be effective and let the rest spill over into the ocean of

Self energy. Our brain cells in particular are excellent at receiving and processing information. Neuroscientists confirm that the right brain nonverbally communicates its unconscious states to other receptive right brains.

In limbic structures of the brain, neural synapses are being created and reinforced by repeated firings. Our capacity for receptivity can be found at the synapses, where there are axons called receivers that branch off the neurons. Branching off other neurons are the senders. These neuronal branches transmit chemical messages between one neuron and the next. These don't actually touch. Between them is a tiny gap, the synapse, through which flow these chemical messages. Joseph LeDoux has said, "You are your synapses. They are who you are."[22]

Although it is intriguing to consider that the essence of our identity is actually empty space through which energy and information is flowing, I think of this synaptic activity as being analogous to a resonant relationship. In this gap between sending and receiving is the possibility of change, of changing who we are, or at least changing our habitual reactions. The receptive, Self-led therapist is also sending information of safety, acceptance, and compassion to the client. The right-brain language of Embodied Self is being received as well. The client's nervous system is receiving that information, which can rewire their habitual relational behaviors. With shifts in the habitual neuronal messages it is now possible for the client's brain (and body, emotions, beliefs, and behavior) to change. Receiving the messages is the key to neuronal revision.

Revision

Shifts happen. The concept of neural plasticity affirms what we experience in therapy. One prominent neuropsychology researcher, Allan Schore, describes the right-brain-to-right-brain process of neural revision. He tells us that the attuned clinician attends to the moment-by-moment nonverbal rhythmic structures of the client's internal state and flexibly and fluidly changes their behavior to synchronize with the client's state in order to establish a safe therapeutic relationship.[23] Safety creates the environment for change to happen in the client's system.

These scientists are affording us a glimpse into the brain and the body of what we are experiencing in our therapy offices during the unburdening step of IFS. When the parts perceive that it is now safe, the hypothalamus releases oxytocin. Oxytocin spurs the prefrontal cortex to send the neurotransmitter GABA to the amygdala. The amygdala is the structure in the limbic brain that activates the part's fearful reaction, and GABA-bearing fibers quell the habitual fear-based response. The bonds between the neurons weaken, allowing for the possibility of creating new synaptic bonds.

The client may see an image of the part letting go of the burden. Or the client may hear the part saying it let the burden go. A client may notice their body is lighter, more spacious, more relaxed. The unburdening process is usually considered as happening only with the person undergoing therapy, but actually researchers confirm that as in any significant relationship—whether it be parent and child, two lovers, or therapist and client—both individuals in the relationship are being impacted on many levels. Scientists tell us that both people's limbic brains are being revised.

In my session with Theresa, she shares with me her shame about her daughter being arrested for shoplifting. I take a moment to somatically resonate with my parts' parental shame and over-responsibility. Theresa seems to feel my presence with her, and her pace of talking is slower, her voice is deeper. In our interactions there are a lot of mindful pauses. Theresa closes her eyes and is quiet for several minutes. I can tell this silence is very different from the times she was dissociating. In these pauses, her defensive protectors have backed off. Her autonomic nervous system has shifted out of the sympathetic state and is in the social-engagement state. In these pauses, she feels the body sensations connected with her shame.

Theresa feels compassion for her daughter and for herself as a mother. She laughs about her wild days as a teenager and feels sympathy for her mother. She has a clear sense of how to support her daughter in this crisis.

Feeling my resonance, perhaps Theresa has oxytocin flowing in her body. Perhaps the GABA-bearing fibers are growing, weakening the synaptic bonds, linking the places in the brain that mediate the qualities and behaviors of parts and Self. Perhaps if we could peer into Theresa's synapses we could know that her habitual neuronal firing pattern has weakened. We could watch new linkages being formed. What we can perceive is that her parts seem to have let go of their fear and shame. They know they are no longer alone in their sense of responsibility. They realize there is no threat in this moment. In fact there is warmth, love, and safety. She breathes it in. When she stays with the part as it experiences wonder and unfamiliarity for the five to twenty seconds required for this new positive experience to register in the brain, new neural circuits of love, compassion, curiosity, and trust can grow. In the days and weeks ahead, as she lovingly engages with her daughter, the synaptic bonds will strengthen from repeated firings, creating new neural circuitries, pathways, and networks that support healthy, resilient relationships.

Has my brain been revised by this session with Theresa? During her silences, I also felt my love for my daughter as well as for Theresa, with warmth in my heart and energy flowing throughout my body. I felt compassion for all mothers and daughters accompanied by a tingling down my arms, spine, and legs, which I feel again as I write these words.

The Practice of Radical Resonance with Wounds of Trauma and Attachment

The Resonant Therapist

I know that any relational interaction goes better if at least one of the persons is more or less in a state of Self energy. As the therapist, it should be me. So I do what I can on my end.

> I am waiting for my client Helen to arrive. I take a moment to feel a vertical flow of energy through my body. I take some moments to check in with my internal world. I find some residues of news on my

car radio and a recent distressing email. I ask that to fade into the background and focus on what I know about Helen. Referred to me by her psychiatrist, who has diagnosed her with depression, Helen has done some reading about IFS and is hoping this model can help free her of her unrelenting fatigue and hopelessness.

Helen and I are about to begin a body-to-body conversation of facial expression, prosody, posture, and movement where both of our inner systems are open to emotional contagion. Resonating with depression and anxiety can be a challenge for me, not to mention diving into the depths of despair. My parts fear I won't be able to help her and we both will feel horrible. They are afraid Helen will sense my fear of her depression. I connect more consciously with my chair and the floor and move my spine a little. I feel more curious than afraid as I rise to open the door.

Helen takes her seat stiffly. She holds her body tensely and she picks at her cuticles as she tells me about her lifelong struggle with depression. She describes the various medications she has been taking and how they have not helped very much, or not for very long. Helen goes on to describe how the depression limits her life, how it is so hard for her to even get out of bed let alone accomplish all she has to do and wants to do. Although she has not attempted suicide, at times she believes death is the only thing that will end this emotional paralysis. She has heard about parts and wonders which of her parts are involved in the depression and if working this way could help her.

I am listening to her words, noticing her body, and noticing my body. I can feel a slight increase in my heart rate. I bring my breath deeper into my abdomen and let it out slowly. I give my fearful part a quick, understanding nod and ask it to sit on my lap and to trust me to sit in the chair. I tune in to the horizontal space around me, remembering I am supported by unseen energies. I remind myself that I just have to be present—that is more important than any techniques. I remember that Helen has Self energy, that, in spite of how it feels to her, the depression is only a part of her, or maybe several parts of her. I feel my heart beginning to open to her. We simultaneously shift in our chairs.

Helen tells me her last therapist was cold and distant, and she is a bit nervous about working with me. I tell her I am touched that in spite of her parts' hopelessness and her bad experience, she has found the courage to come today. I notice a whisper of a part wanting to be a better therapist than the last one that is willing to back away. I tell her I trust we can help the parts with the depression, and that we will start with listening to where the depression is in her body.

Finding, Focusing, and Fleshing Out Parts through Resonance

Helen turns her attention inside to find the body sensations that feel like the depression. She finds a crushing heaviness in her chest that makes it hard to breathe in. She also notices a tightness in her belly. She points to her diaphragm area. I am surprised at her interoceptive ability, especially considering her depression diagnosis. I synchronize my breath and allow my chest and belly to slightly mimic those symptoms. After a few moments, though, Helen goes blank. She says she is afraid she is not doing well, that she is stuck. I feel a bit blank as well, a vague feeling in my head. I remind my part we've been stuck many times and it always works out. My head feels clearer.

I say to her, "Let's just get curious about this blankness. We don't need it to change. Let's keep it separate from the fear and try to just be with it. Do you sense this blankness somewhere in your body?" Helen sits across from me with her eyes tightly closed, trying to notice the blankness.

Continuing to listen to my body as I notice hers, I feel some anger coming up from my belly. I don't feel angry at Helen, and I'm pretty sure I'm not angry about anything else. I wonder if I am feeling something that Helen is not yet ready to notice. If it is Helen's anger, I wonder if it is a separate part or another aspect of the blank part. I wonder if she is mad at me for not preventing this uncomfortable stuckness, or if the anger is covered up by the blankness.

SM: Helen, let's go back to the sensations in your chest and belly. What is it like now?
Helen: My chest feels heavy. It's like it's trying to squash the tightness in my belly.
SM: How does your belly respond to that?
Helen: Now my mean part is coming up. Sorry.

> SM: Let's welcome all of these parts. They are coming up quickly. To keep track of them all, how about if you find some objects in the room to represent them.
>
> Helen finds a blanket for the blank part, and other objects for the part that fears the blankness, the heavy heart part, the tension in her belly part, the mean part, and the one that apologizes for the mean part, placing each one on the floor.
>
> SM: Walk around all these parts now. As you do this, maybe your body will tell you which part you want to focus on.
>
> Helen is most interested in the blank part represented by a blanket because she thinks that has to do with her depression.

Developing a Resonant Relationship with a Part

You may recall that the question that facilitates a Self-to-part relationship is "How do you feel toward the part?" When I ask Helen to feel the blanket, to hold it, to find out how she feels toward it, she answers, "Compassionate." I don't sense compassion when I look at and listen to Helen. I wonder if she is really in touch with this quality or if she had just learned from her reading that this is the "right" answer.

> SM: Where in your body do you feel this compassion?
> Helen: I actually feel blank toward it.
>
> This tells me the blank part is blended with her.
>
> SM: Let me speak to the blank part: Would you be willing to back off a bit? We won't try to get you to stop blanking out her feelings, we just want to help you with your job, and for that we need a bit more of Helen to be present.
>
> The blank part separates enough for Helen to feel some curiosity toward the blankness. I suggest she show her curiosity to the blanket. She picks up the blanket again and examines it.
>
> SM: How does this blank part feel toward you?

Helen: The blankness doesn't believe I can take care of myself. She thinks I'm a young girl who needs its protection.

SM: Step away from all these objects on the floor. Come over here and stand next to me.

From this place in the room, Helen can see that she is not the blankness, not the part the blankness thinks she is, nor is she any of the other parts represented by the objects in the room.

She is now differentiated from the blank part and can begin to establish a resonant relationship with it. She moves toward the blanket representing the blank part and strokes it, telling it she is not the young part that it thinks she is, but she can help it take care of this young part if it is interested. She tells me she has a sense of this young part that the blank part is trying to protect. She feels a cold knot in her stomach. She sees a little girl, about five, sitting all alone on her bed in her room. When she tells me she feels compassion toward this little girl, this time it feels genuine. We now develop a resonant relationship with this young girl. Helen lets the girl know she knows how cold and alone she feels. She tells me the part is looking at her hopefully.

Witnessing the Part

SM: If it is OK with her, you could go into her room and sit next to her on her bed.

Helen goes into the room and sits on the bed next to her part. We find another object to represent this young part and place it at Helen's side.

SM: Invite her to show you or tell you what she wants you to know.

Helen: The little girl is looking up at me. She looks so sad. She looks frozen and frail and can't speak.

SM: Yes. So maybe your body can give you a sense of what she wants you to know.

Helen's body tightens up and she feels colder. She feels like she can't move. I put a blanket around Helen as she sits in my office. Helen tells me this is what the depression feels like at its worst. Helen lets the little one know she really can understand how it is for her. I find another blanket for Helen to put around the object at her side.

The girl still isn't talking, but Helen talks to her. She tells her she isn't alone right now. She lets her know it's OK if she doesn't want to talk. Helen feels warmth in her heart toward her, and she tells her she will keep her warm and will be happy to help her in any other way. The little girl lets her get close enough to snuggle in with her and rests her head against Helen's breast.

Helen tells me she has told other therapists about this "inner child" and her family's history as Holocaust survivors, her father's addiction to alcohol and drugs. She has worked on her eating disorder, and how her mother would cook huge amounts of food on the Sabbath, encouraging everyone to eat, then in private would criticize them for eating too much. She believes her eating has been an attempt to take care of this little girl's neediness. She feels like this little girl's story has not been so deeply felt before. I have had many clients who have told their stories to other therapists, but their parts never really felt heard. The memories of their wounds are mostly right-brain, and they need the right brain to get them. When the right brains of the client and the therapist are both resonating, the effect is compounded.

Unburdening

In the next couple of sessions Helen continues to develop a resonant relationship with this five-year-old girl. It is easier for Helen to focus on her without blanking out. This protector seems to have transformed into a "blanket" part to warm the little girl.

Helen tells me the little girl has taken off the blanket, is leaving the bed and moving around her bedroom. She is relaxed and smiling. Helen's body is also more fluid and relaxed. The five-year-old tells Helen she is ready to leave her bedroom and come into the present with her. She leaves her frozen fear and sadness in the old house. Helen tells me she senses the girl moving around the office, exploring the objects we have placed in the room to represent Helen's parts. Helen looks content. She smiles and looks into my eyes. I smile back and feel warm tingling throughout my body. With the five-year-old safely present with us we have a clear path to work together to heal her legacy of trauma and her eating disorder.

Radical Resonance with Attachment Wounds

Wounds of attachment are addressed brilliantly with IFS. The client's Self is the primary agent of healing attachment wounds with the young part, supported by the therapist's Self. In IFS the job of the therapist is not to meet the exile's needs, but rather to avoid a part-to-part relational dynamic that will perpetuate the attachment style. The Self-led IFS therapist creates the conditions for the client's Self to heal the wounds of the vulnerable part and create a secure attachment with this part.

The practices of Somatic IFS, especially the practice of Radical Resonance, offer a right-brain approach to connect with the abandoned, neglected, and traumatized parts in the fullest sense possible. A resonant relationship can heal the wounds of attachment. Whether the client's parts have adopted anxious, clingy behaviors or distancing, avoidant ones, underneath their behaviors they are longing for connection. Because of their history of a lack of secure connection, the client's parts are adept at sensing the therapist's emotional availability. Often the attachment wounds occur long before verbal language has developed to be able to communicate physical or emotional needs. If the infant did not have attuned parents who are "children whisperers" their vulnerable parts may want the therapist to meet their unverbalized needs. In Somatic IFS we become "body whisperers."

Patricia had a hard start in life. Her mother was date-raped at sixteen and dropped out of school to raise her daughter as a single mother. Her mother's parents helped her financially but not emotionally; they blamed Patricia's mother's "wild" behavior for her rape. Patricia came to therapy because her insecurity was driving away the women she was in relationship with. Women would get involved with her sexually, but then they would get distant and leave or would cheat on her. Afraid and anxious when she was alone, Patricia would desperately hang on to a bad relationship. She blamed herself for these failed relationships but didn't know what to do to keep these women in her life.

At first Patricia's parts that experienced neglect were completely blended and no Self energy could be found. Understandably, her mother was overtaken by her own parts during the crucial times of

Patricia's development and she was not available to form a reso-nant connection. Patricia's inability to bring her Self energy to her neglected parts communicated her experience—there was no one at home, often literally as well as metaphorically. Patricia relied on me for emotional regulation, acceptance of her parts' needs, and con-fidence to provide what is needed until her parts would be able to allow her Self energy to emerge.

We find the controlling, demanding, and desperate protectors and give them appreciation and compassion. There are many times when I feel a lack of connection with Patricia as her parts cut off from me. At those times I struggle with boredom and frustration. I am able to tolerate the pain of disconnection when I consider that my response is my resonance with her parts' stories. Whatever neuronally based protective strategies Patricia developed in her embryonic stage are now being expressed in her posture, facial expressions, gestures, muscular contractions, breathing patterns, and sexual energies, and they are being transmitted in my body and mind. I find compassion when I remember that Patricia's protective parts are trying to keep her spirit from being annihilated.

Patricia's protectors come to understand that their strategies are doing the opposite of what they intend. After addressing and gaining the trust of the first rung of protectors, I resonate with ones they pro-tect—the parts that had been left alone while her mother worked, the parts that suffered when school friends asked where her father was, the parts that fear she has inherited the badness of her father. I feel a strong pull on my heart and some waves of righteous anger when hearing about her experiences.

Patricia starts to believe she deserves to be loved. She becomes better at attending to her own neediness and loneliness. She begins a new, healthier relationship. She is sometimes able to reassure and comfort her fearful parts when her partner leaves town. Her impul-sive behaviors lessen. But she still often feels anxious and untrusting in this current relationship. Talking about the stories of her mother's unwanted trauma-induced pregnancy have not helped reduce the anxiety. She fears that her need for reassurance could drive this woman away too.

It is important for me to join Patricia in the dark watery realms of her original attachments to her mother, in the womb where there was the trauma of the violation and where she sensed she was not wanted. Through the umbilicus Patricia may have sensed some withholding of life-giving nutrients and energies, some revulsion toward her as she took up space in her mother's body. Although Patricia's memories of this time are entirely in implicit memory, her experiences were influencing her developing limbic structures and would become the soundtrack of the relational challenges in life.

Since Patricia has no conscious memories of the time of her trauma, she has to imagine it. We go to her body before her birth to venture into the dark watery beginnings. I guide Patricia to imagine connecting through her umbilicus to her mother's uterine wall. She imagines herself as that embryo who relied totally on her mother for her life. She places her hand on her belly and breathes in through her navel. Her body contracts in flexion and she rolls onto her side. Her body feels dead, dull, empty. She curls up more tightly. She begins to sob and tremble.

Over the next several sessions we return to this place of her earliest attachment experience through her umbilicus and the embryological structures that are the precursors of her nervous systems and organs. Each time, Patricia resumes the fetal position. Sometimes she lies stiff and inert in that position, and at other times she sobs and shakes. Eventually she relaxes and unfolds and rests on the floor. She imagines receiving nourishment and loving energy from the earth—energy that is free from trauma and shame, energy that is rooted in the same core that nourishes and supports all of us. I feel moved to tears. When she connects through her navel to this universal energy, she feels relaxed, calm, and "floaty." Patricia is more able to bring her Self energy to her parts both when she is alone and when she feels insecure in her relationship.

These sessions with Patricia, viewed through the neuroscientific lens articulated by Daniel Siegel, demonstrate that somatic practices activated the regions of Patricia's brain between the limbic structures and the middle prefrontal cortex that are involved in the neuronal resonant circuit. In other words, these practices provided a bridge between the areas of her brain that were unconsciously determining her parts' protective strategies and the conscious part of her brain that can restore emotional regulation, resilience, self-awareness, and compassion.

We all have secure attachment that can be uncovered as parts are unburdened. Even the most extremely wounded parts have not given up on getting what they need. Unplanned pregnancies, substance abuse during pregnancy, rape, or domestic violence—these are unfortunately all-too-common situations for mothers and the embryos growing in their bodies. Intrauterine relational ruptures can be far-reaching. Birth traumas, abandonment at birth, and negligence are some of the occurrences in early life that require a resonant approach for their healing.

Healing Relational Ruptures

So far we have focused mostly on how to form resonant healing relationships, but what about when there is a rift? Relational ruptures are inevitable. Knowing that these breaks to a resonant flow are part of the relational territory rather than a catastrophe, my parts relax a bit. I don't like ruptures happening, but it helps to remember that they are inevitable. I also remind myself that they are quite possible to heal. Like broken bones, relationships get stronger in the place where they broke. If the relationship is important enough, both people will be motivated by the pain to find a way to mend the rift.

The inevitable relational ruptures we encounter are explained by neuroscience. The information about our adaptive brain and nervous system through Siegel's interpersonal neurobiology and Porges's polyvagal theory helps me normalize these ruptures. I have learned that when our parts perceive a threat, because of the DNA inherited from our hunter-gatherer ancestors, our autonomic nervous system goes into a state of either mobilization or collapse. Generally speaking our clients don't threaten our life. But when the process is so stuck that we feel dumb as dirt, when our clients point out our inadequacies, our parts hijack our resonant capacity.

I understand that the other reason we fail to sustain this resonant state is, ironically, because of the hard-wiring that enables us to be resonant. When our clients are blended or flooded with parts with extreme burdens, our nervous system—our right-brain limbic structure—in fact, our entire body—reverberates with and mirrors the fear, anger, despair, or shame. It takes a couple seconds before the mind is assigning blame and our heart closes down. Our Self energy is off-line. Our reactive state is conveyed quite eloquently through our body. Our clients are at least as good as we are at reading nonverbal signals. Their lives have depended on it. We could be heading for a parts-led relationship where the roles of perpetrator, victim, or savior are center stage and where the actors' roles can switch quite suddenly.

We all have parts-driven habitual responses to relational ruptures. We all have burdens from breaks that did not heal. We carry sadness, anger, despair, confusion, and fear from unresolved conflicts that led to abandonment or even physical wounding. Our parts' initial impulses might be to defend, to pull away, to avoid, to minimize, to blame ourselves or the other person. Our client may not be willing to work with us to find a way through the impasse. If they simply quit therapy, we feel abandoned. We feel vulnerable. Perhaps our professional reputations are on the line.

When it is a therapeutic relationship or any other relationship with a discrepancy of power, it is appropriate that those of us whose role has more power tend to the client, or the one who has less power. We may need to get outside support to work with and unburden our parts before we have enough Self energy to begin the repair process.

Whether it is a professional or a personal relationship, if we do attempt to find a way through the impasse, we can expect our parts will be reluctant to step aside to allow for a Self-led repair. Often the rupture was caused by parts, and they are still hanging out on the corner, ready to defend their territory against the enemy. My part's version might sound like "Do you think I didn't hear you? Saying it again and again, louder each time, isn't working for me." "Oh, *you* don't feel heard yet? Well, *I* don't feel heard either, and I was the one who brought it up, and now you expect me to forget about my needs and listen to yours?"

If I can look underneath my outrage and defensiveness, often I find a part that is hurt by how the person is characterizing me (selfish or inconsiderate, for example). My more vulnerable parts are worrying that if I can't defend myself against this judgment, how worthy am I to be in this relationship? I may lose this person who is so important to me.

If I can slow down long enough to be with my protectors' automatic defensiveness, I may be able to be with the physical sensations. I may be able to focus on my closed heart, my rapid heartbeat, my shallow breath. I may be able to ask my parts, "Are you sure you want to keep this going? You do know where it is heading, don't you?" My parts answer, "YES WE DO!" as my fists clench. If I can ask again, I may be able to stop escalating and take a pause. I might remember I have a lot of practices and skills that have been helpful in the past. I feel how bad I feel, how unpleasant and stuck this present moment feels. I consider I may be able to do something to head things in a different direction. I bring a sliver of awareness to my breath. I breathe into the pressure pushing down on my sternum. I breathe into the tension in the back of my neck. I breathe into the tightness in my belly that is restricting my inhale. I may be able to look at the face of my "adversary." She may look unappealing at first. I look deeper and see there mirrored a similar fear, sadness, and uncertainty. My heart melts a tiny bit. With that little bit of melting, like our polar ice cap, everything else begins to melt as well. Together we find a way to flow into our usual coherence, sharing our vulnerability and coming to a deeper knowing of each other.

If we can remember our true nature is juicy, that our body after all is two-thirds water, the momentary rigidity of our protectors trying to keep our ego intact can dissolve. With a repair, the relief and joy we feel is like that of a baby in games of peek-a-boo or hide-and-seek, or when the baby is tossed up in the air and caught a second later. What was rent in the fabric is now whole. The rewoven threads of connection are more precious to us because of our fear of loss, the pain of disconnection.

Cultivating Our Resonant Capacity

Cultivating and embodying Self energy is a lifetime endeavor. I have come to appreciate that my most challenging clients have helped me find parts that may not have otherwise shown up. Since the practice of resonance requires the body to be a resonant vessel, the therapist can explore parts that fear opening to being deeply impacted physically, emotionally, and energetically. Most of us have been hurt in relationship, and those wounds not yet healed will be shaken loose as we open to the reverberations of our wounded clients.

Most of us have walled off our soft, impressionable body and mind as a protection, and our parts can come to realize that our body—our breathing and our cellular and organic processes—knows how to take in and let go. The optimal functioning of our relational brain has never been more crucial to our survival. Coming decades will require even more resilience.

We bring our body fully into our relationships with our clients, offering our body as a vibrational vessel of healing. With compassion for our own human limitations we speak from our heart, encouraging other hearts to open to their flowing power. We wade into the relational waters and sense the depths, the temperature, the hidden currents, whirlpools, or rapids. The client's inner system is communicating its unconscious states nonverbally to our receptive right brain even as we keep our head above the emotional waters. As we attend to the moment-by-moment nonverbal rhythmic structures of the client's internal state, we flexibly and fluidly synchronize with our client's state. The sensitively attuned parts of the client's system sense the possibility of a safe, healing environment.

The client's protectors relax and allow the vulnerable parts to feel held in a safe, compassionate relationship. Their stories of trauma, neglect, and abandonment are dropped like pebbles into calm, clear waters; the ripples recede at the shore. The stories between and behind the words, the stories not yet ready to be shared, the stories hidden deep in the interior of the primitive neurological structures, are sent in energetic frequencies into the relational field. Our heart and our entire body receive and reverberate with the tremors of this somatic, energetic communication. Our heart-felt, radically resonant receptivity is transmitted wordlessly and received vibrationally by the client's bodymind system.

The following exercises cultivate our capacity to resonate with the reverberations of others' implicit stories. With the first exercise we move into relationship from our heart, and the second exercise helps us shift our habitual listening and responding patterns. With the next three exercises we revisit and embody our earliest attachment experiences from the blastocyst stage to the embryonic and birth process to reconnect with our innate capacity for nourishment, protection, connection, and differentiation. We revisit the three layers formed as the embryonic cells multiply, migrate, and differentiate, organizing into three vertical layers, each layer offering what the developing organism requires for its survival, growth, and development. Reconnecting with each of these layers, we experience our capacity for nourishment, for protection, and for differentiation as well as any obstacles to these innate resources. Encountering parts as we explore these layers, we can release the burdens of our earliest attachment injuries, which are the root of later parts' relational burdens. As we restore our body's inherent resonant ability, we become a vessel for revising relational wounds.

Radical Resonance revises and transforms both the therapist's and client's internal systems toward more fully embodied Self leadership. In a state of Embodied Self our energetic and vibrational alignment allows us to recognize our functional unity with other beings. We experience our interdependence with all of life and come to realize what Daniel Siegel calls "the deep reality that we are a part of a larger whole." Radical Resonance provides a safe container for exploring and potentiating the final two Somatic IFS practices, Mindful Movement and Attuned Touch.

EXERCISES

Moving from the Heart into Relationship

PURPOSE   To bring qualities of Embodied Self energy established with vertical alignment into relationship; to move into relationship from the heart.

INSTRUCTIONS:

The first two steps of this exercise can be done individually, the last two with at least one other person in the room. Take as much time as you need with every step. Pause to notice body sensations and feelings, to spend some time either enjoying the experience or exploring any blocks to it, to find parts and give them what they need.

1. Connect with Below and Above: Standing or sitting, focus on your bones, from the small bones of your feet upward through

your pelvis, spine, ribs, sternum, and cranium. Make any shifts to allow these bones to feel supported from below. Imagine being rooted like a plant through the floor to the earth. While rooted, can you also float upward? Feel into the space above you and around you, and breathe that spaciousness into your body. Feel or imagine a flow of energy traveling through this vertical line from the core of the earth to the farthest reaches of space.

2. Move into the horizontal plane: As you move, frequently pause for moments of awareness. Explore your relationship with the space around you as you move in any direction, in any position. Invite your curiosity about your inner system to lead your movements. Notice if you can maintain your vertical alignment as you move into this horizontal plane; if not, take a moment to re-establish it.

3. Move into the relational realm: Expand your awareness to include others in the room. Notice if there are parts that want to connect with others and parts that don't. Breathe into your heart, sensing its place along your vertical line. Invite your heart to lead your movements. If your heart draws you to connect with another person in the room also moving from their heart, let your heart lead you as you consider how to express this connection nonverbally—either with or without physical contact.

4. One option for physically connecting is back to back, either standing or sitting. Take some time for both people to adjust to size differences, to get comfortable, to feel their backs touching each other, each maintaining their vertical alignment. Yield into the contact. Notice the sensations, the movements; experiment with other movements. Experiment with sounds—humming, vowel sounds, feeling the reverberations. Play with this way of relating, noticing the relational dynamics.

REFLECTIONS:

1. In pairs, take turns sharing what you noticed during the first two steps, including resources and obstacles, as you established vertical alignment and then shifted into the horizontal plane.

2. How did you both choose to connect? How was it different to have your heart lead the way?

3. How did your relationship evolve regarding communicating, leading, and following?

4. How are you feeling now within yourself and toward the other person? Did your vertical alignment change the ways you related?

5. Is there anything from this experience to take into your relationships with others?

Developing Receptivity

PURPOSE This group exercise develops resonant capacity by practicing expanding habits of listening beyond receiving the verbal content to include nonverbal language, one's own bodymind inner experience, and information from the Field of Self energy.

INSTRUCTIONS:

1. Form groups of five people. Each person will have a task and the tasks will rotate, with one speaker and four listeners, each listener attending to a different mode of receiving the flow of energy and information from the speaker. The timekeeping will be shared by the group and strictly adhered to by passing a clock to the speaker at the end of their time. The listeners may want to take brief notes.

2. The speaker faces listener 1 and speaks for three minutes about a topic of their choosing.

3. Listener 1 focuses primarily on the verbal content of the speaker's story. Listener 2 focuses on the nonverbal language of the speaker. Listener 3 attends to their own inner bodymind response. Listener 4 is open to receiving information from the Field of Self energy, even if it seems irrelevant.

4. Each listener reports for one minute on their listening experience.

5. The speaker responds for one minute.

6. Rotate roles.

REFLECTIONS:

1. When everyone has had a turn, each participant reflects on the experience as a listener. Which role felt most familiar, most enjoyable, most difficult, most surprising?

2. Each participant reflects on their experience as speaker being listened to in four different modes. Did you feel resonated with? Did you find one listening focus to be most facilitating of resonance?

3. Is it possible to listen simultaneously in all four ways?

4. Which of the foci/tasks do you want to integrate more into your listening habits?

Embodying the Embryological Roots of Our Resonance

The first steps of these next three exercises can be done individually; the latter ones require a partner.

Resonating from the Front Body

Our earliest attachment experience involved the front body. From this front body the umbilical stalk grew and attached to the uterine wall. This embryonic layer morphed through various forms to become our organs of digestion and elimination.

PURPOSE To reconnect with the innate capacity of the embryo for safe and satisfying attachment and nourishment by embodying the front body of the embryo and the developing endoderm, the source of our gut wisdom.

INSTRUCTIONS:

1. Bring awareness to the front of your body. Brush your hands from your face to your feet. Move through space from your

front body. Begin to notice what particular qualities you find in your front body. Allow those qualities to be expressed in your movement.

2. Bring your hands to your navel. Feel your breath moving your navel in and out. Remember or imagine how you grew a stalk, reaching toward the womb and firmly attaching either to your mother or to the core of the earth. Through this connection you receive all you need, physically and emotionally. Through this umbilicus you can also let go of any parts' burdens you absorbed, sending them back through the generations.

3. Receiving all this nourishment, your body grows and develops a tube, your gut tube that goes from your mouth to your anus. You are now free to detach from the watery womb and emerge onto land.

4. As you move on land—standing, sitting, or lying—stay connected to your gut tube. Bring awareness to your lips, your tongue, mouth, esophagus, stomach, intestines, anus as you move through space, aware of any differences in how you perceive your environment.

5. Notice others in the room. You may have a "gut sense" of who, if anyone, you want to partner with. From your front body, move toward that person.

6. Move together, each from your front body, from your gut tube. Notice the quality of the movement. With this layer of innate ability for nourishment, is it easier or more challenging to be impacted by your partner's experience?

7. When it feels right to share verbally, take turns speaking and listening to each other from the front of your body.

REFLECTIONS:

1. Name the qualities you first noticed as you moved from your front body. Are these different from the qualities you usually feel as you move through the world?

2. Name any feelings, sensations, images, or thoughts that arose as you attached through your navel. What nourishment did you receive? Did you release any personal or intergenerational legacy burdens from your time in the womb?

3. How is your "gut wisdom" different from your intellectual wisdom?

4. As you related with another from your front body, nonverbally and verbally, how was it the same as or different from your usual way of relating? How was it to speak from your front body? To listen from your front body? To what degree were you willing to be impacted by your partner's experience?

5. What did you learn about your own bodymind system from this relational exchange?

6. Are there people or situations where you feel relating from your front body would be beneficial?

Resonating from the Back Body

As the back layer formed, it sent out an embracing protective membrane that became a fluid-filled amniotic sac, eventually becoming our skin and nervous systems.

PURPOSE   To reconnect with the innate capacity of the embryo for protection and safe connection by embodying the back body of the embryo and the developing ectoderm.

INSTRUCTIONS:

1. Bring awareness to the back of your body in any of these ways: let your breath come into your back, move your spine, touch the back of your body from top to bottom, lie on the floor on your back, ask a partner to touch the back of your body, stand back to back.

2. Standing, move from the back of your body. View others from the perspective of your back body. Notice what sensations, emotions, qualities arise. Parts? Protectors? Exiles? Self?

3. Remember or imagine your back body growing a protective membrane that surrounds you entirely, attaching to the wall of the uterus. You may want to find a blanket to wrap yourself in to help you remember this protection. Feel yourself held securely in this safe, protective sac, bathed in the womb's waters, free to become who you are.

4. This back body layer also forms a tube that eventually develops into your brain and spinal cord. It also becomes your skin and other organs of perception.

5. When you feel ready to leave this watery world of safe connection to emerge onto land, find a way to bring this intrauterine protection with you. Bring awareness to your skin, your spine, your brain, your senses. Feel how these structures protect you today. Standing, sitting, or lying, move through space from your back body, aware of any differences in how you perceive your environment.

6. Notice others in the room, and see if there is an openness to connect with another. From your back body, move toward that person. Move together, each from your back body—spine, skin, nervous system. Notice the quality of the movement. With this layer of protection and differentiation, is it easier or more challenging to be impacted by your partner's experience?

7. When it feels right to share verbally, take turns speaking and listening to each other from the back of your body.

REFLECTIONS:

1. Name the qualities you first noticed as you moved from your back body. Are these different from the qualities you usually feel as you move through the world, or from moving from your front body?

2. Name any feelings, sensations, images, or thoughts that arose as you provided this protection. How did your parts respond? Vulnerable parts? Protective parts?

3. How do your skin and nervous system protect you today? How else do you provide your bodymind system with necessary protection?

4. What differences did you experience perceiving, moving, and relating from your back body?

5. How was it to speak from your back body? To listen from your back body? How does your back body affect your willingness to receive and resonate with your partner's experience?

6. What did you learn about your own bodymind system from this relational exchange?

7. Are there people or situations where you feel relating from your back body would be beneficial?

Resonating from the Middle Body

At about four weeks after conception the middle layer formed, integrating the front and back layers. This middle layer eventually becomes the mesoderm: skeleton, muscles, connective tissue, heart, blood vessels, kidneys.

PURPOSE   To reconnect with the many creative possibilities for connection and differentiation by embodying the middle layer of the developing embryo.

INSTRUCTIONS:

1. Bring awareness to the middle layer of your body, where your front and back bodies meet. Draw a line with your hand from the top of your head down through the side of your body, imagining this layer throughout your body.

2. Lie on the floor on each side, becoming more familiar with this layer. What are some of the qualities you sense of this middle layer? Do you sense its ability to weave and connect the front and back layers while also staying separate?

3. Standing, move from the middle of your body. This layer connected your entire body as it developed into your bones, muscles, and fascia. Move from your bones. Move from your muscles. Move from the fascia that embraces and connects everything and gives you shape.

4. Another organ that developed from this middle layer is the heart. Sense into your heart powerfully and diligently circulating blood to every cell, as a field of energy far stronger than the brain, as the subject of love songs and poetry.

5. Let your bones, muscles, and heart move you toward a partner. Your connective tissue encases and separates each body structure and also is the path of communication and connection. Feel your separateness as well as your connection with your partner.

6. Together with your partner, with stillness and silence, words and movement, through your front, middle, and back bodies, explore your connection. Is it possible to interact from all three layers simultaneously, from your gut, brain, and heart?

7. Join another dyad to form a group of four. Three people choose one layer each to resonate with the fourth person. The fourth person speaks or moves for three minutes while each resonator responds from front, middle, or back body. Rotate roles and discuss.

REFLECTIONS:

1. Name the qualities you connected with in your middle body that were different from the front and back. Which of the three are more familiar, more habitual for perceiving, moving, speaking, and listening?

2. Name any feelings, sensations, images, or thoughts that arose as you connected with your middle body.

3. How do these systems that develop from this embryological layer—the bones, muscles, connective tissue, and heart—facilitate resonance?

4. As you related with your partner, each one of you exploring each layer, fluidly moving between them and integrating them, what did you learn about your bodymind system?

5. How was it to listen with your gut, heart, and brain all together? Did you move between them? Is one more familiar?

6. What are the gifts and limitations of each layer? How do they work together to help you resonate? Are there people or situations where a particular layer of your embryological body facilitates greater ability to be impacted by, to resonate with, and to revise another's implicit story?

5

Mindful Movement:
Restoring the Flow

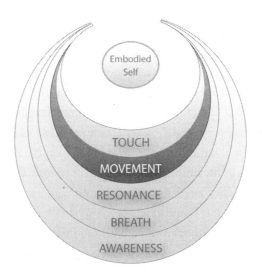

"*MOVEMENT?*" A THERAPIST MIGHT say. "I can skip this chapter. I don't do that." Most therapists and clients assume that they will sit parked in their seats for the duration of the session. Even many Dance Movement therapists tell me they typically sit with their clients for much of their sessions. Sitting and controlling our movement impulses is one of the many social norms that govern our behavior and lessen social anxiety. We have learned from our early experiences in school to override our impulses to express our curiosity, our excitement, and our fear through movement. Instead we sit quietly and we move only when granted permission, and then usually only in a prescribed way. There are labels for those children who struggle to adapt to these expectations. Over the years we have developed many ways to control or ignore our impulses to move until it has become second nature.

And yet there are health consequences from too much sitting and from stifling our natural movement impulses. Movement is a primary way for emotions to be expressed, to be known, and to find a path to flow toward release. The practice of Mindful Movement can uncover the dormant impulses to move and can safely restore the flow of our emotions and of our life force.

And we don't have to leap around the room. When I introduce this practice in a workshop, some participants look at me with hesitation. Movement may have been a source of shame and ridicule. They may have been pushed to excel at dance or sports. Their protector parts want to avoid a repeat of exposing their inadequacies. These participants breathe a sigh of relief when I invite them to begin by simply lying on the floor. In the stillness, the busyness of life drops away. They begin to trust the support of the floor below them. They begin to notice the subtle movements occurring in their body. They become aware of a movement that wants to happen. They might find the movement opens up a pathway for eventual healing.

Movement is the primary way we express our emotions. The Latin root of the word "emotions" is *emovere* (to move out). Charles Darwin, in his seminal book *The Expression of the Emotions in Man and Animals,* concluded that we human beings, like many animals, express our emotions through movement: subtly through a sneer, smile, squint, or clenched jaws, or more obviously by running, embracing, striking out, or playing dead.[1] Unlike animals in the wild, humans have parts that fear they will be judged or rejected for expressing their emotions and so bury their feelings and manage their movements. Yet the emotions will look for a way to "move out."

Our body is part of this moving world. The sun, moon, rivers, oceans, clouds, trees, grasses, animals—all are moving at various speeds, in various cycles, in spirals and waves. When we stop our frenzied, driven activities, we notice the rhythmic pulsations of our heart and our breath. We notice digestive rumblings and slight muscular fasciculations under our skin. We might feel like we want to lie on the floor forever. We might curl up on our side or roll around on the floor. Like yin and yang, one phase of our inner dance has within it the emergence of its opposite. We open to life and novelty, and then close to rest and restore. We expand and condense, fill and empty, flex and extend, contract and relax. We move toward, we reach out. We move away, we recoil. As we are mindful of the gross and subtle ways our life energies are flowing, as one movement gives rise to the next, we discover parts whose stories may best be told through movement.

We move in the womb and we never stop until we breathe our last breath. Our motor skills develop throughout our life span. At every age, our emotions, intentions, beliefs, needs, and desires are expressed through movement and fuel motor development. The early movement patterns begin in the womb and develop rapidly during the first year of life. Movements of side lying, head righting, rolling, belly crawling, hands and knees crawling, and finding a way to sitting, standing, and walking form the foundation for more complex movements. When movement is unrestricted and integrated, life flows freely.

In between conception and death, however, we encounter many situations—physical and emotional—that can interfere with our motor development. If we lack secure attachment, certain movements are perceived to be dangerous. We may not have been able to move toward or push away from a parent whose behavior is unpredictable. Our own natural pace of motor learning may have been interfered with by parents' anxious or controlling manager parts. Early trauma may have interrupted our natural unfolding by trapping our developing bodies in an exhausting cycle of overactivation and immobilization. Interference or interruption in our motor development affects our perceptual, cognitive, and social development as well as our lifelong movement patterns. Bringing awareness and an invitation to the story of blocked motor development offers a path for healing and restoring the flow.

The stories of interrupted motor development from the earliest beginnings through childhood are waiting for someone to listen. Vulnerable parts are bursting for their stories to be heard. Movement may be the only channel. They may want to show us their attempts to reach out, to cling, to push away. Their locked-in feelings want permission to move out, to sequence through the body to completion. When the exiles' emerging energies threaten to overwhelm the system, protector parts step in. Protectors use nervous jiggling, extreme sports, sexual acting out, and, at the most extreme end, suicide and homicide to distract from the exiles' stories or to attempt to soothe or discharge pent-up energy. Protector parts can also commandeer fitness movement practices to manage images, which cultivates competition, performance anxiety, perfectionism, and mindless repetition. Protectors may express hostility as fingers poke at the air or hands slap the body. They use the horizontal hinges in the body that are made for movement—the jaw, neck, back, hips, knees, and feet—to stop the free flow of expression. At these joints the protectors block the impulses to kick, to run, or bite, suck, scream, or speak, to express joy, curiosity, sexual energy, excretion.

The parts' interrupted movement story can lie stagnant for years in frozen postures and faces, repetitive gestures, and chronic pain and stiffness. Somatic IFS therapists invite awareness to movements—and lack of movement—because both are the outer manifestation of the client's inner world. Clients stroke their face or hair, hug their body, touch their heart, shrug, turn away, and hunch their shoulders toward their ears. We invite mindful awareness to these movements. When they lead to the untold stories of parts, we find, focus, and flesh out the parts. When it seems a movement story has been blocked, we initiate a subtle movement to free it up. Welcoming and witnessing movement allows the story held in the tissues to unfold.

I got my first glimpse of the usefulness of Mindful Movement as a bodyworker when my efforts to help fifteen-year-old Jason with his shoulder pain were not working. I stopped working on his tissues and asked him when he first felt this pain. He told me that another boy had made him angry. "Did you feel like hitting him?" I asked. "Oh, I would never do that," he quickly responded. "Yes, of course, but did you *want* to?" "Well, yeah!" he replied. "Just show me, really slowly, how you would have done that."

Jason took a stance, made a fist with his right hand, drew back his arm, and slowly allowed the spiraling movement to flow from his shoulder out through his fist. As he was able to complete the interrupted movement impulse, the tension left his back. He walked away with a satisfied smile. From this experience I learned that a sensation of pain or numbness could be a sign of an interrupted movement impulse to strike out, to reach toward, to push away, or to rest. As the movement story is told and witnessed, the ease and flow in the body is restored.

Movement, done mindfully, also helps us cultivate Embodied Self energy. There are many movement practices—such as the many forms of yoga, self-defense, martial arts, and dance—that support all the qualities of Self energy. They promote mental clarity, calmness, and focus. They help relieve chronic stress patterns and increase body awareness. Somatic IFS encourages clients to develop a regular movement practice to support and further their healing process. It is important to consider that our parts will co-opt any of these practices to accomplish their protection roles. They use spiritual practices to avoid emotions. They can take jogging or exercise to an extreme. They can practice *asanas, katas,* and choreographed dance movements from an attitude of competition or perfectionism. When these practices are adopted by parts, they might interfere with the client fostering their Embodied Self energy.

Attending a national women's martial arts conference, I was admiring the powerful, flowing, expert movements of the experienced karate and aikido practitioners. Not being an expert martial artist myself, I took my sore, tired body to a workshop that offered a more free-form expression of movement. As I began to move to the music and the leader's guidance, I saw that many of the other participants continued to move through the room as if they were defending themselves from invisible attackers. They seemed to be at a loss to allow their movements to flow from their inner urges, from the music, the environment, or the group energy, and so they fell back on the habitual, choreographed *katas*. This saddened me and left me with a resolve to invite participants to bring mindfulness to their movements to notice if there are parts rehearsing habitual patterns. The energy in the room changes as the participants experiment with unfamiliar movements that often surprise them.

Why *Mindful* Movement?

Mindful Movement specifically avoids reenacting the traumatic experience. Somatic IFS differs from a purely cathartic approach to trauma therapy. The stories of trauma that are frozen in the body need to thaw gradually through mindful, moment-by-moment witnessing by Embodied Self energy. When the client touches into the traumatic memory, movement fueled by intense emotion could result in flooding or re-traumatization. Careful somatic tracking guides the pace of the expression. The movement story—from the first attempts to escape to safety, to the adaptive reflexes to fight or flee, then to the collapse when the body's resources are overwhelmed—can be slowly and safely revisited.

We bring mindful awareness to the impulses to run or fight and initiate gentle movements to the collapsed or numb areas of the body. Mindful Movement can restore the truncated responses, physically contradicting the overwhelm and helplessness of the event. Bessel van der Kolk in *The Body Keeps the Score* explains that the medial prefrontal cortex, which he refers to as the "watchtower," is the area of the brain that deserted trauma survivors during the trauma, and it needs to be brought back online.[2] Mindfulness engages this area of the brain and leads to changes in this and other regions related to body awareness and fear. Movement is one of the practices he recommends for facilitating body awareness and strengthening the body's system for regulating arousal.[3]

Mindfulness creates the conditions for Embodied Self energy to be present with the parts as they make themselves known. It ensures the part won't repeat the traumatic experience of feeling overwhelmed and alone as it attempts to retrieve its painful story out of the archives of memory. The therapist does not encourage the client to relive the entirety of the emotionally distressing experience but instead attends to emotional regulation in the client's system. Parts may strive to take over the system with their energies and their emotions, eager to demonstrate their urgency and their pain. Parts whose stories of pain have been suppressed and exiled often try to throw a coup. They may want to flail, kick, punch, scream, curl up, run away, or otherwise fully express the extent of their pain in hopes of discharging the strong energies. Without a witness to their story, some parts pump the carburetor of emotions while others push on the brake pedal until the system is flooded.

Without the presence of Self energy, there is a danger of the client's system being re-traumatized. Without careful consideration of the ecology of the inner system, there might be a protector backlash that will slow down the healing. The part's movement story is mindfully witnessed, digested, and integrated into the whole bodymind system. Movements done mindfully are often slow and subtle but also can be large and expressive. The key is *mindfulness*, which allows for the Self energy of the resonant embodied therapist and, in time, the resonant embodied client to hold the part's expression. Mindfulness creates the conditions for the movement to be an agent of transformation for the client's limbic brain and body systems.

What Movements Are We Mindful Of?

As with all the practices, the therapist begins with awareness of themselves, knowing that their inner state is communicated to their clients through their movements, even the subtle movements of their eyes and facial muscles. Worry, judgment, boredom, frustration—all are communicated through movement and posture, as is compassion, presence, and acceptance. That emotional states influence postures and movements has been observed by Hippocrates, Charles Darwin, and William James, and now via functional MRIs. Our language expresses this close connection between movement and emotions. The words "attitude," "posture," and "stance" have meanings that refer to both mind and body. Does the therapist feel imprisoned in their chair, or by the computer screen? When sitting, does the therapist feel free to allow their energies to move their spine, shoulders, arms, and head from their grounded pelvis? Simply shifting the sitting posture can often immediately restore the flow of Self energy through the body. The resonant therapist may notice movements or impulses to move that are coming not from their internal system but from the dyadic relational field. The therapist may unconsciously mirror the client's movements or realize the inhibited movements of the client are looking for expression in their movements.

181

The therapist is also noticing the client's movements and can then decide whether or not to invite the client's mindful attention to the movement. Observing the client's hand spontaneously curl into a fist, the therapist could name what they notice and ask the client if they notice it as well. The client can deliberately repeat the hand flexion while noticing any emotions, images, thoughts, or memories that come up as they slowly flex and open their fist, possibly leading to a part. This decision and many others involve the "art" of therapy and are informed by the practice of Radical Resonance.

The therapist can invite movement with every stage of the IFS process. When a part first shows up as an emotion or a thought, movement can flesh out the part more fully. Often the client's words hold clues to their parts' movement stories that want to unfold. The client may speak of feeling stuck, paralyzed, or torn, or trying to cling to, push away from, wiggle out of, or strike back. When words and thoughts lead to a dead end, embodiment through movement may be the way forward. We might invite the client to move to differentiate from a part, to demonstrate the part is retrieved from the past, and to embody the unburdening process. Movement can help with the integration phase. There may be a posture, gait, or gesture, some freed up impulse that represents the change. The movement repeated over time can reinforce the change. At the end of a powerful session, I often suggest to a client that they walk around the block with these qualities before they get behind the wheel of their car. Walking and other cross-lateral movement patterns reintegrate the brain and nervous system and reorganize the mind–body connections. And the unburdening process continues as the client moves through their life, and it often leads to uncovering more burdened parts.

We also bring mindfulness to the movements that help us find and sustain Embodied Self energy. The ongoing natural movement in our body echoes nature's cycles. We find movement even in stillness. When we get quiet enough, we discover an entire symphony of rhythms. The rhythmic filling and emptying of our breath lulls us. The blood beat of our heart has a faster tempo. We might notice fluids flowing in our digestive organs. If we are quite still, we may notice the subtle long, soft waves produced by cerebral spinal fluid being released and absorbed in the brain and spinal cord, gently dragging the bones and fascia along with them. The constantly shifting vibrations and the often unheeded faint drumbeats reconnect us with the natural rhythms and movements of our living body. Our body may want to lie in stillness or may move us in ways that surprise. The dynamic, fluid state of Embodied Self energy in movement can become a wonderful practice.

Mindful Movement Is Associated with the Fire Element

Fire has been an important part of cultures and religions from ancient times. The Greeks associated the element fire with energy, assertiveness, and passion. Fire brings heat, light, growth, and purification. In tantric yoga the qualities of fire are found in our physical, energetic, and emotional bodies and influence the personality. Centered in the appropriately named "solar" plexus, this energy center, or chakra, is linked with the digestive tract. Our digestive system transforms food into the fuel to move forward in the world.

The heat from fire increases movement in molecules; movement in turn creates heat. Movement produces a large proportion of the body's heat. At this moment, even as we sit in relative stillness, a coordinated and orchestrated movement within each cell and among all the cells makes up the process that provides us with the energy to sustain life. When we move, of course, we require more metabolic fire. This metabolic support is provided by food that is converted into glucose and sent to the tiny cellular structures called mitochondria that combine it with the oxygen we have breathed. This process supplies the energy needed to maintain a slow burn. Tense muscles that hold chronic tension require just as much metabolic support as do our moving muscles. Releasing the muscle tension makes more energy available for moving forward toward our life goals.

On an emotional level, our internal fire is expressed in joy and laughter as well as passion and anger, and all these emotions are expressed through movement. Protector parts may exile any of these emotions to keep the system safe. The force of emotionally fueled movements can eventually erupt despite the best efforts of protector parts. Just as fire that is raging out of control can cause serious damage, mindless movement can be dangerous. Experts in forest management use controlled burns to cleanse our forests of underbrush so that wildfires are not so devastating and to abate greenhouse gases. Mindful Movement provides a controlled burn to the pent-up emotions and behaviors.

Fire, like movement, is transformative. Fire transforms water into steam, wood into ash, and mud into stone. Transformations are a seemingly magical process. The transformational power of fire enthralled me as a clay artist. I selected the dried pieces that were to undergo the trial by fire and recycled the rest. We placed small clay figurines representing gods and goddesses of fire as we tended the firing of the kiln. When the kiln finally cooled down, we excitedly opened the door to behold the altered pieces. The glazes were now molecularly bonded to the clay body, the dry mud of the pieces now permanently transformed to a stone-like structure, similar to the way that pressure and heat from the depths of the earth change mud to stone. Now, as a Somatic IFS therapist, I am privileged to witness the transformative effects of Mindful Movement.

Body Systems Associated with Mindful Movement

The Muscular System

Our internal system affects and is affected by our muscular system, and our muscular system affects our movement. The skeletal muscles are the prime movers of the body as they act on the joints to move the body. From the smallest muscle in the body (the stapedius, which tenses the eardrum to muffle our chewing noise) to the large quads and hamstrings that propel a runner to cross the finish line of the Boston Marathon, muscles have three options. They can shorten, they can lengthen, and they can lock down. All of the actions, postures, gestures—the entire spectrum of movement possibilities—are defined by these three possibilities.

Muscles define our size, our shape, and the quality of our actions. The muscular system is made up of more than six hundred individual sacs or compartments that function as a whole system with many parts, similar to our internal system of parts. No one compartment of muscle acts independently of the other compartments that relate to its function. They all work in an enormously complex collaboration. Deane Juhan in *Job's Body* suggests we think of the muscular system as one muscle with millions of fiber-like cells that pull in different directions as some of them contract while others extend. A flaccid core requires a tight lower back; a sagging chest tightens the back of the neck.[4] The interaction of the muscular system to create balance may have its source in the interrelationships within the individual's internal system acting on the muscles.

Emotions affect muscle tone. When the muscle tone is too high, the body appears tense, wound up, rigidly held, or bound. To the touch the muscles feel stringy and hard, like beef jerky. Movement may be effortful, controlled, or constricted. When the muscle tone is too low, muscles are flaccid. The tissues feel soft, slack, lifeless. The body appears lethargic, passive, lacking the energy to move. There may be an imbalance of muscular tone in the body, with some muscle groups hyper-toned while others are hypo-toned. When muscle tone throughout is even, the body is alert, relaxed, and ready. The flesh feels firm but pliable. The muscles can move with a graceful, easy, coordinated, harmonious freedom, and both posture and movement will signal Embodied Self. Our muscular system, as well as our internal system, needs to strike a compromise between stability and freedom.

Somatic educator Mabel Elsworth Todd connected muscle tone with psychological issues in 1937 in her book *The Thinking Body*. This book is considered to be a classic study of the physiology and psychology of movement and was an important part of my bodywork education. She wrote, "Unbalance of this special tone function is often the accompaniment of neurotic disturbances . . . which physical exercise alone does not serve to correct."[5] She describes how every thought and emotion is accompanied by a muscle response, and eventually the responses become fixated in our postures and gestures, as unique as our fingerprints. In this way our parts' burdens become recorded in our posture and movements. Our beliefs in our unworthiness, our criticisms, our feelings of shame, despair, loss, and fear become embedded in our muscle imbalances. Todd tells us that because these imbalances are habitual and familiar, they tend to not register consciously. Bringing mindfulness to our gait, posture, and gestures reveals the underlying muscular patterns and the associated thoughts and emotions.

The Autonomic Nervous System

Although all the body's systems are functionally interdependent, the autonomic nervous system (ANS) is intricately and intimately linked with the muscular system, in addition to the actions of most of our other bodily systems involved in movement. How we move through the world is guided by our ANS—whether we move away from, move toward, freeze, or collapse. Our posture and movement are a reflection of the activity of our ANS.

We now understand Darwin's treatise on emotions and movement in animals, as well as Todd's perspective on the influence of emotions on human movement, from Stephen Porges's pioneering polyvagal theory. Porges has helped us understand that the actions of our ANS are part of the inheritance for our species' survival, with significant practical implications for clinical work with trauma and the practice of Mindful Movement. Polyvagal theory offers a path to reframing the adaptive trauma responses, to releasing the trauma responses of the ANS, and to restoring the capacity for healthy relationships through mindful expression of the movements mediated by the ANS.

This theory concerns the actions of the two parasympathetic responses of the ANS when faced with a threat, based on the two separate branches of the vagus nerve. The vagus nerve is the longest nerve in the ANS. Its dorsal branch originates in the brain stem and wanders into the stomach and intestines. It is the more evolutionarily primitive part of the parasympathetic branch and lies in wait as a last resort. The ventral aspect of the parasympathetic branch is the most recently evolved structure of our ANS and is found in humans and other mammals. According to Porges, when perceiving a threat we first utilize this ventral vagal system. We reach out to interact, to be rescued, to be soothed, to feel safe.

In response to trauma, we travel through the evolutionary history of our ANS. Calmly walking along, we encounter a challenging situation, such as meeting someone in a dark alley who we fear might hurt us. The initial movement impulse directed by our ANS is our most evolutionarily recent, the ventral vagal "socially engaged" state to call out or reach out for assistance. When it is clear that no help is available, the next recently inherited response kicks in. Our sympathetic nervous system takes over, mobilizing us to respond to the threat by either running away or fighting. Our body releases hormones, our heart rate spikes, blood is rerouted to our large muscles to ready them to help us escape or stand and confront the situation. When we either get away to safety or realize there is no threat, our sympathetic state downshifts and the ventral vagal branch is back online. Our parts that mobilized around the threat are not traumatized.

Trauma occurs when both ANS functions have failed. Our ANS resorts to the most primitive response from the dorsal vagus nerve, the one we inherited from our reptilian ancestors. The dorsal vagus nerve inhibits the sympathetic branch of the ANS. Facing an inescapable threat, we freeze, collapse, and dissociate, just as many primitive animals do. We physiologically and emotionally shut down. This long nerve affects many systems of the body, such as the limbic brain, the heart, lungs, and digestive organs. Our body releases more pain-killing endorphins that numb or dissociate us. Our muscles become limp and flaccid, blood pressure takes a steep dive, the heart slows. The mind and the sensory organs become numb, and memory access and storage are impaired.

I again refer the reader to Deb Dana's *Polyvagal Theory in Therapy*,[6] referenced in the third chapter of this book regarding the theory's application in Conscious Breathing. Her descriptions of noticing and naming bodily experiences apply as well to movement as they do to breathing to assess the state of our ANS. Through this process of recognizing the movements, postures, and gestures that indicate which branch is dominant—the sympathetic branch or the dorsal vagal part of the parasympathetic branch—we can regulate our automatic responses and shift the states of our ANS.

Influences on the
Practice of Mindful Movement

Hakomi

The mindful exploration of our habitual, largely unconscious gestures began with a question from the late Ron Kurtz, who developed the experiential, body-centered psychotherapeutic method of Hakomi: "Is your thumb stroking your finger or is your finger stroking your thumb?" I soon realized that the intention of this question was the invitation to bring mindful awareness to our movements as a path to our core emotions and beliefs.

My Hakomi training taught me to pay attention to the movements my clients make as they talk. I began to notice movements I had previously disregarded—shoulders sagging, raising, and shrugging, head turning away or reaching forward, arms vehemently slapping the chair, and legs jiggling. I noticed my clients' hands were very active—touching cheeks, covering lips, clutching hearts. Hakomi invites mindfulness to these naturally occurring movements and supports their expression in order to reveal the unconscious core beliefs that are organizing the client's behavior. I learned to consider these movements as additional communication beyond what clients were telling me verbally. Sometimes the movements seemed to support the words, and other times to contradict what was spoken.

At first I feared that my clients would feel self-conscious and exposed, but I discovered that in an atmosphere of loving presence, inviting mindful exploration to these largely unconscious gestures allowed clients to contact their unmet needs for soothing, their fears of being seen or heard, and their beliefs about not belonging. My clients were willing to experiment with the movement—to exaggerate it, to slow it down, or to do an opposite movement. Often movement became the path to meeting the need, calming the fears, or altering the core belief.

Dance, Yoga, Martial Arts

Other movement practices that have shaped my body and mind, as well as the development of Mindful Movement, include dance and various forms of yoga and martial arts. One tai chi teacher suggested that the precisely choreographed sequence of moves that we were practicing began with one person moving with such authenticity and grace that his neighbors began to mimic the movements, which, generations later, became formalized into the tai chi or chi gung movements we know today. He had us observe the movement of the wind in the trees and a cat who often joined our class as the real tai chi masters. Inspired by his words, and recognizing that specific movement practices can facilitate mindfulness, I developed a practice that coordinates walking, breathing, and arm movements as we intentionally connect with earth and sky energies flowing through the body. I have introduced this to several clients. So far, I have one follower! Every week we start the session with this walking meditation, and it helps us both be more present and grounded for the rest of the session.

Authentic Movement

In Authentic Movement the client tunes in to their inner-world thoughts, feelings, images, and sensations and allows the movement to emerge from their inner experience. The client's movements are witnessed by an attuned therapist, and the experience is processed together. IFS and Dance Movement therapist Susan Cahill describes this process as similar to employing the practice of Radical Resonance explored in the previous chapter: "Being seen as the mover or seeing as the witness become interchangeable positions during the practice. In each position there is an attempt to see or witness oneself clearly as both mover and witness."[7] My experiences with these teachers and colleagues, my academic study, and my clients and students have convinced me that movement—moving with mindfulness—is an essential component of Somatic IFS.

Polyvagal Theory

Again I appreciate my friend Deb Dana for helping me understand the application of polyvagal theory to the resolution of trauma, which has influenced the practice of Mindful Movement in Somatic IFS. As explained earlier, when trauma is not resolved, the effects from the ANS activation are trapped in the tissues. The physical and emotional effects depend on whether the person's ANS is primarily stuck in sympathetic or dorsal vagal parasympathetic activation, or oscillating between the two.

The biochemical residue from sympathetic activation leaves a person restless, mistrustful, hypervigilant, and anxious, vulnerable to serious health problems if the state is prolonged. Their eyes may dart around the room, their arms and legs held tightly or jiggling. A trauma survivor exhibiting the dorsal vagal state of shutdown feels despairing and isolated, locked in paralyzing terror. They typically blame themselves for failing to avoid the trauma, or even feel guilty as if they caused it. Physically, hormones are held in the body; digestion, sexual energy, and immunity are suppressed. Many chronic health problems may ensue also when this state is prolonged. The client's face may look vacant or frozen; stuck in a dorsal vagal state they may be low energy with their posture collapsed, unexpectedly fall asleep when you get close to the trauma, and have trouble hearing or making sense of what is said to them.

The polyvagal view of the various ANS responses to trauma is that these responses are instinctual and adaptive for our survival. This perspective is a relief to clients burdened by shame and blame for their actions and nonactions. We bring compassion to the physical expressions of sympathetic activation. With the part held in a safely connected relationship, the trapped movements are mindfully expressed and witnessed. Movement allows for a release of the fear and anger held in the body and lets the ANS return to a ventral vagal state. A client whose ANS is chronically in a dorsal vagal state, or whose recall of the overwhelming event activates this state of shutdown, is reassured that their collapse, their dissociation, and their numbed emotions are beyond their control. This state, like the sympathetic activation, is a result of our evolution as a species. Because predators don't eat prey that appear to be dead, feigning death is an autonomic legacy that has permitted our species to survive.

As the client understands the adaptive nature of their physiological response, the path is clear for re-storying the trauma through movement in order to restore the physiology. This path is a reverse of the sequence of the ANS during trauma. The path to healing through movement is to move back through the succession, starting with the frozen state, revisiting the sympathetic state, and finally restoring the ability to find relaxation, peace, and connection.

With a client chronically in the dorsal vagal freeze response, we bring mindful awareness, acceptance, and welcome to a more explicit embodiment of their physical state. The client may curl up in flexion or become listless, collapsed, frozen. With the multiplied awareness of mindfulness of both client and therapist, the frozenness begins to thaw. The therapist supports any movements and can offer an invitation to imagine or even experiment with a small movement. The client often feels some awakening of sensation in their limbs, like a tingling or trembling. The therapist encourages these movements, reassuring any parts that this is a path to healing. Therapist Peter Levine, a longtime friend and colleague of Porges, has studied the shutdown response through animal observations and bodywork with clients. In *Waking the Tiger*, he explains that emerging from shutdown requires a shudder or shake to discharge suspended fight-or-flight energy.[8]

Moving out of this numb state, a person can expect that the suppressed mobilization of their sympathetic activation will show up in movement impulses to hit, to kick, to run, to recoil, to push away—any of the movements that had been inhibited by the dorsal vagal branch of the ANS. In these movements we can read the story of the attempt to defend against or to escape from the danger. The therapist directs the client to bring mindfulness to these impulses and invites the movement to be expressed in a way that allows the client to be present to the feelings associated with the movement. The therapist frequently slows down the pace of the automatic sensorimotor activity, keeping the focus on the movement and checking to see that the client's Self energy is present to the parts as the story unfolds. Freeing up the movements associated with fight and flight, *with mindfulness*, allows the client to have a bodily experience of successfully navigating the threat. It provides for an embodied re-storying of the trauma. The parts can let go of the beliefs about their helplessness and unworthiness, their feelings of shame and fear and despair. A somatic unburdening occurs as the accumulated metabolic waste products in the muscle fibers are released and other physiological processes return to homeostasis.

Mindful expression of the sympathetic activation allows the ANS to return to the ventral vagal parasympathetic state. The parts previously frozen in time and space—and in the physiology—have been unburdened. The client and therapist feel connected with each other and with the unburdened parts. The client may sigh, yawn, stretch, and continue to shudder as additional tension is shaken off. Over time the client will experience fewer extreme oscillations between shutting down and reactively mobilizing, will more easily track their own ANS responses that fluctuate throughout the day, and will more easily return to the ventral vagal state.

As trauma is resolved through Mindful Movement, each of the states of the ANS operates in a dynamic, balanced way. Sympathetic activation provides power, creativity, alertness and concentrated focus for tasks and activities such as dance, sports, play, artistic expression, or writing. When the ANS needs a bit of recovery, the dorsal vagal state allows the client to momentarily "space out" or rest in stillness. When relaxing or playing with loved ones, the client enjoys the ventral vagal aspect of the parasympathetic branch. The client, through co- and self-regulation, learns to move fluidly along these three states of a restored healthy-functioning ANS: sympathetic, dorsal vagal, and ventral vagal.

Body-Mind Centering

Body-Mind Centering (BMC) has been a more recent influence on the practice of Mindful Movement. During my bodyworker years I was first drawn to this embodied approach to movement and consciousness developed by Bonnie Bainbridge Cohen. I appreciated the psychophysical and developmental principles and the experiential approach that uses movement and touch to repattern the bodymind. Bainbridge Cohen makes the analogy of the body being like sand and the mind being like wind blowing on the sand. Observing the body's posture and movements gives us a window into the emotions and beliefs of the mind. In her work with clients, she initiates movements to effect changes in the bodymind relationship.[9]

Bainbridge Cohen's protégés Susan Aposhyan and Lisa Clark have applied her teaching to psychotherapy and yoga, respectively. Through their teaching I have explored how our inner systems are the outgrowth of the seeds of our earliest movements, which lay a foundation for the future development of our body and mind. Linda Hartley, also a practitioner of BMC, tells us, "Through movement the fetus' nervous system develops, awareness of itself and its environment begins to emerge, and a foundation for future learning and modes of interaction and response is established."[10] BMC considers that any delay or disruption in the natural unfolding of motor development can affect later movement patterns, which often correspond with disruptions in emotional and cognitive development. This movement practice of Somatic IFS accesses parts associated with the disrupted movement patterns and offers them a restorative experience, affecting the entire bodymind system.

The perspective of BMC considers parallels between the forms of embryological and infant-developmental movement patterns (ontogenetic) and the evolutionary progression through the animal kingdom (phylogenetic). Normal movement development follows a sequence that in some ways parallels evolutionary development. Susan Aposhyan writes, "As human infants progress from infancy through the first year, culminating in learning to walk, we recapitulate the basic patterns used by progressively evolving species for locomotion."[11] Along with other psychologists and psychomotor and somatic educators, BMC recognizes parallels in cognitive and motor development between humans and other species, evident in the developmental stages of human embryos that resemble those of other species such as fish and birds, and Aposhyan's Body-Mind Psychotherapy looks at the psychological aspects of these stages of development.

Lisa Clark has applied Bainbridge Cohen's lifetime work to yoga that considers the embryological basis of various structures of our body that become the template for our perceptions, movement, and psychophysical expression. Through her guided movements I have re-experienced emerging from my watery beginnings to become a land-based creature, sensing the origins of my neurocellular patterns and my endocrine system, fluids, and organs. Particularly illuminating for me, as a Somatic IFS therapist who assumes that Self energy is present within our body from birth, is the realization that these qualities are exhibiting themselves even at conception. As the single fertilized egg rapidly divides, fluid moves between the cells and the extracellular matrix. These pulsating movements result in new structures forming in the embryo as it organizes along a vertical line. By revisiting these early structures through movement we can access the source of our inherent Self energy.

The embryological structure that lines up at the front of this vertical organization is the yolk sac, which provides the rapidly growing embryo with all the nourishment it needs. This front body soon grows a stalk attached to the uterine wall that becomes the umbilicus, then morphs into the soft gut tube from mouth to anus, and eventually becomes the organs of digestion and elimination, what we consider the endoderm. The back body at first forms the amniotic sac, which embraces the tiny being with a protective shield, which in time becomes the spine and the nervous system and then the skin, which make up the ectoderm of the human body. So we have within us, within the first weeks after conception, from the front and back structures, all we need for nourishment and protection, and our body continues to develop in complexity to provide those crucial needs. Later burdens can cause our parts to believe we need to seek anywhere but within for nourishment and protection, and these burdens will result in no end of relational quagmires. But through embodying these early structures and their movement patterns, we revisit these early templates to connect with our Embodied Self energy and our inherent qualities of creativity, collaboration, and resilience. The movements of the embryo become the building blocks of locomotion.

BMC considers five sequential and interrelated movements that begin in the uterus and become the prototypes of our later physical and emotional development. The more basic the action, the more it influences the later psychosocial cognitive development. Bainbridge Cohen teaches that the movements of yielding, pushing, reaching, grasping, and pulling begun in the uterine fluids as the embryo is attached at the navel are the foundation of both physical and psychological development. These sequential movements occur through the six limbs of our body—the head, tail, two arms, and two legs. The navel is at the center. The limbs all originate from this central core. Floating in the amniotic waters, the embryo plays with these five movements, preparing for its emergence onto solid land. After birth and for the rest of our life we reach out with the sense organs of our head, with our pelvis, and with our arms and legs. The reaching out may involve more than one sense or limb—for example, reaching out with the mouth and the right arm to say hello and shake a hand. Or both arms to hug. Polarized parts may show up, such as a reach through the arms while the lower body pulls back. The free flow of these movements from or through our limbs can be blocked or inhibited by wounds of trauma and attachment.

Through a BMC lens I observed the movements of my first granddaughter from birth through her childhood. Searching for the breast with her nose and mouth she pushed and reached along her vertical axis. She gained increasing control and coordination over the gross movements of her trunk, legs, and arms. She pushed down on her arms and navel as she reached upward with her upper trunk and head. Eventually she was able to coordinate her push and reach through her limbs with her spinal twists to roll over. As she learned to sit up, the sitz bones of her pelvis became an additional source of grounding (assisted by a fluffy diaper).

Over the next few months my granddaughter learned to support her newly integrated spinal core upon all four limbs. Then, really ready to rock and roll, she scooted across the floor with her arms dragging her lower body to explore the electrical outlets and the rickety plant stands. Her movements at first mimicked frogs, then lizards, and eventually the contralateral movements of mammals. The crawling patterns that I observed, initiated by yielding weight into and pushing out from the ground, according to BMC, are facilitating her ego development and a boundaried sense of self.

She reaches toward the coffee table with both arms and pulls her body upright. Bending her knees and looking down, she wonders how to get back to the earth. I am in awe of her determination and passion. I know that all of these movements are crucial to developing her perceptual relationships, including spatial orientation and body image, and the basic elements of learning and communication. She is experiencing through movement a sense of being a unified whole, with separate parts that are both differentiated yet connected.

Restoring the Flow
through the Five Movements

Integrating all these movement theories and practices into IFS has been at the core of my work with clients, consultants, and workshop participants. With clients who have experienced trauma and attachment wounds in utero or infancy, working with the internal family in an embodied way offers an opportunity to enter the preverbal matrix of the parts' experience directly. The earliest attachment wounds can be healed through imaginary movement, beginning with the ovum's journey through the fallopian tubes and continuing through gestation, and by revisiting the stages of motor development. Burdens inherited or energetically transmitted intergenerationally can be cleared. These "legacy burdens," as they're called in the IFS model, can be released through movement.[12]

IFS recognizes that certain qualities are "lost" when a part absorbs burdens. These qualities in very young parts are embedded in the body's systems. Motion, as well as emotion, wants to sequence through the body. Movement wants to flow to and from the ends of each of the six limbs. All the types of movements desire expression. With traumatic wounding these resources get restricted, truncated. Protectors inhibit movement impulses, freezing the body story. The stories of interrupted motor development are evident in the truncated movements. We invite and support these movements to restore the resources that are our birthright. As the early movement patterns are reenacted, the associated memories and emotions may be accessed, allowing for witnessing and unburdening of the parts.

In Somatic IFS workshops, my students enjoy playing one-celled creatures, starfish, jellyfish, snakes, frogs, lizards, and finally mammals. We begin with *yield*, which is, surprisingly, often the most challenging of them all. Yielding reveals our relationship with the earth. It involves a surrender, a letting go, a state of being rather than doing. It requires trusting, being receptive to support. Many of our parts resist yielding. They prefer to do something—to keep moving so they don't get stuck. They don't trust resting into the ground. Some participants rediscover the nourishment of this state of being and feel as if they could stay in this state forever. Others feel the impulse to curl into a fetal position, held supportively in this posture in order to reengage with their internal rhythms. Their skin becomes the cellular membrane as the body breathes in and out, surrendering to the earth below and pulsating with the rhythm of the earth. They feel their body breathing in and out. They connect with their navel and revisit the powerful moment of their first attachment to the wall of the uterus to receive life-supporting nourishment that travels to head, tail, and each of the limbs.

The energy from the nourishment gives rise to the impulse to push against the earth, the first expression of a separate sense of self. The movement of *push* affirms a right to a boundary, our right to claim a separate identity, our relationship to the space around us. They rise up into space and reach from the navel through the top of the head with their eyes, nose, mouth, lips, tongue. This vertical line of energy connects the organs. The head connects to the heart, the heart and lungs to the stomach, spleen, liver, gall bladder, pancreas—as well as the glands, bones, and muscles of the upper body. They connect with the third, fourth, fifth, sixth, and seventh chakras and the movements and emotions connected with these energy centers. They play with flexion and extension and twists of the lower spine to experience a vertical line from navel to tail with the movements of yield, push, and reach, connecting the organs, glands, and other body structures and energy centers of the lower body between the navel and the tail, or pelvic floor.

A full *push* leads to the impulse to *reach*. When the movement of reach is supported by the foundation of earth and sky, we don't overextend. When we have claimed the power of our separate identities, we have the courage to reach for what we want and need. With this movement we explore our world. As we reach for what we need or want, we *grasp* it and *pull* it toward us. As *reach* involves extension, *grasp* and *pull* involve flexion. With the movement of *grasp* we hold on to what we have sought. We claim the value of the object or person for us. The movement of *pull* draws it into close proximity, such as to the mouth or the heart where it can be used or treasured. Reclaiming our power to reach, grasp, and pull allows us to release the energy of flexion. When this sequence feels complete, the cycle can begin again as the body organically shifts into a state of *yield*.

Tuning in to the navel, the participants imagine themselves to be a six-limbed starfish as they explore pushing and reaching from their centers to their limbs, and they enjoy the freedom of their spine as they play at being vertebrate species like the fish and snake. They mimic the homologous actions of a frog, moving simultaneously both arms, both legs. With yield, push, and reach they crawl like lizards on the floor, alternately extending and flexing their sides in homolateral movements. The diagonal, contralateral movements of mammals often lead to an impulse to stand and walk, completing the stages of movements from conception to the first year of life. Through these playful movements, the participants repattern their own early developmental experiences.

As participants re-embody the basic developmental movement patterns, they discover the places where their development was hindered. The block may show up as a difficulty with the movement—a weakness, a lack of integration or ease, a disconnection from the movement. It may show up as emotions, or feeling nauseated, or feeling distracted or dissociated. They mindfully explore the movement until they feel a release or a change, a restoration of the ease, flow, and grace of the movement. We take many mindful pauses for awareness and for integrating the experience before they explore the next developmental stage.

From this vertical connection from navel to head and navel to tail, they connect each of the other four limbs to the navel, and to each other through the navel. The movements of push, reach, grasp, and pull through each of their awakened limbs allow for wiggling, rolling, crawling, and maybe even sucking of thumbs as the movements reflect both ontogenetic and phylogenetic movement development and the emotions embedded in these movements.

Case Examples of Mindful Movement

The following summaries of client sessions demonstrate the integration of the many influences on the practice of Mindful Movement: the five foundational movements and embryological approach of Body-Mind Centering; the mindful exploration of habitual postures, movement, and gestures of Hakomi; and the application of polyvagal theory with trauma. Each example shows how injuries at important developmental periods cause movements to be lacking in integration, how these disruptions interfere with people's moving forward in the world, and how Mindful Movement can restore the flow.

Early Developmental Trauma

Thea's relational trauma began at conception. Her fifteen-year-old mother lacked the emotional, social, and financial support to raise a child. Despite not receiving the necessary emotional, energetic, and physical foundation before birth or during her childhood, Thea survived and in many ways thrived. But she was drained from her decades of over-functioning. Her hard-working managers were up against a wall—not able to keep going but terrified to trust that Thea would be OK if they rested.

As Thea gets in touch with the exhaustion, she feels how difficult it is to even sit upright. After initial reluctance, she gives in to the impulse to lie down on the floor. As I guide her to yield to the support of the floor below her, she lies there for a long time. Eventually her body begins to relax, and her breath to deepen.

Thea: My lower arms and hands are tingling.
SM: Stay with these sensations of tingling in your arms and hands.
Thea: There is a lot of energy in my arms.
SM: Notice if the energy in your arms wants you to move.

Thea begins to push against the floor with her arms.

SM: Let this movement stay small. Just slowly lift off from the floor an inch or two, noticing how it feels. Come back to yielding into the floor, then when you are ready, come back to pushing . . . just slowly and mindfully back and forth from yielding and resting to pushing. What do you notice?
Thea: My arms feel strong. It feels light and easy as I rise up. And it feels good to have the floor below me as a support. My lower body relaxes more. It's like it is reassured of my core strength, my resilience.
SM: Continue with this, letting your lower body be aware of your strength and resilience as you push up from the ground.

Thea comes to all fours and plays with yielding and pushing from her upper and lower body, and eventually reaching through her head and her tail. Thea discovers that yielding is different from collapsing, which her hard-working managers fear. Yielding into a safe connection had been interrupted from the time of conception and throughout her childhood. She lacked the foundation for the next developmental movement of push, and she struggled with differentiating from her mother. Now able to yield and push, Thea is energized by pushing through every limb. Mindfully experiencing the movements of yield and push allows Thea to experiment outside of session with ways to trust in the support available to her and to assert her needs and her autonomy in relationship, so she can continue her important work in the world without getting depleted.

Relational Ruptures

The movements of push and reach in my session with Maya demonstrate how mindfulness of these movements led to a relational repair. Maya had a conflict with her sister that resulted in her sister cutting off from her. She feared that she and her sister were reenacting patterns they learned from the behaviors of their mother toward their aunts. Maya was concerned that she and her sister might pass these patterns on to their own children. She hoped Somatic IFS could help her release these patterns through her body.

Maya goes inside to feel what her side of the conflict feels like. She feels the strength of her defensiveness.

Maya: If I didn't push her away, I'm afraid she could take away my entire reality. This fear is in my diaphragm. It's a hard lump.

As she speaks, I notice a slight forward push of her right shoulder.

SM: Stay with this hard lump in your diaphragm. See if you notice anything happening in your shoulder.

Maya's shoulder pushes forward, slightly at first, and then becomes larger and aggressive, soon involving the whole right side of her body. Her face has a determined set.

SM: Is there a part connected with this movement?

Maya: Yes, it's a part pushing my sister away. I'm letting my part know I like its strength. I know it has been trying to protect me. But I don't think this part knows it has also pushed my sister away.

With her words, the movements become smaller and eventually quiet as her arm rests in her lap. Maya feels a warm, melty place in her heart that cares about her sister and desires a healthy connection. She feels the energy from her heart flow through her shoulder and her arm toward her sister. The lump of fear is able to sequence from her diaphragm to her shoulder and her body as she expresses her power to protect herself. Reassured of her power, with the release of the lump in her diaphragm, she can access the energy of her heart. The pushing movement in her shoulder transforms to an impulse to reach out to her sister. The sequence of movements from push to reach from her heart leads to a resolution of the rupture with her sister.

Eating Disorders

My session with Lori demonstrates how she resolved through movement a paralyzing "push-pull" tug-of-war regarding her eating. One part had pushed her to lose thirty pounds and get off all her diabetic medication. Another part of her was trying to pull her off the brink of the success of these healthy behaviors. We gave each part a chance to move and talk.

Lori stands up and faces where she had been sitting and speaks from the pushing part: "I made her lose weight. I was afraid she would die." With pushing gestures she admonishes Lori to shop, cook, eat the right foods, and exercise.

Then the other part pulls her back onto the couch. Lori speaks from this pulling part: "I'm afraid too! I'm terrified of Lori being healthy and living her life more fully. The pushing part is exhausting me with this crazy strict health plan. We will probably gain the weight back and feel like a loser."

Lori finds respite from this paralyzing polarization in the movement of yield. She stands up to feel the floor beneath her feet and begins to walk slowly around the room. At first her gait is stiff and hesitant, and then it becomes freer. She finds a sculptural object on my altar. She says it represents Life. She reaches for it and holds it close to her heart. She looks at it with tenderness. Tears begin to flow down her face. She feels in her heart her desire and commitment to be in alignment with behaviors that support a healthy life as represented by the sculptural object, and it is from this place that her arms reach, grasp, and pull toward her heart what she desires.

Lori returns to the couch. She feels relaxed and calm, and more confident she can move toward healthy behaviors in a more relaxed way. I am deeply moved by Lori's capacity to embrace life, knowing that her family system included debilitating physical and mental illness and suicide. We both acknowledge how challenging it is to change entrenched behaviors. She knows the right foods to eat, and she says that choosing those foods feels as dramatic as having to change a switch in her brain. She understands it takes some time to rewire her brain, and that when she makes good choices, not from a pushing part but from her Self, she is forging new connections that eventually reduce the pull to eat the wrong foods. To anchor this newfound embrace of life, she borrows the object from my altar so she can practice reaching for it, grasping it, and pulling it toward her heart.

Chronic Physical Symptoms

Blocked emotional expression resulting in chronic painful jaw tension and a debilitating TMJ disorder led Debra to seek Somatic IFS therapy. Debra had suffered for most of her childhood from a life-threatening illness. Not wanting to trouble the people she sorely depended on, she held her feelings inside.

As Debra experiments with moving her jaw in various ways, she starts to feel angry.

Debra: Now I am remembering when I was in the hospital. I see a five-year-old. She is standing in her hospital bed, holding onto the cold bars. She is angry with her mother for leaving her alone.
SM: As you sense her anger, what do you feel in your body?
Debra: I feel a big lump in my stomach. It feels stuck there.

I notice her jaw clamps shut.

SM: Focus on the lump in your stomach and let's see if we can help it move.

Debra: I feel like I want to bite, but I don't want my anger to hurt my mother. She has done all she can for me.

I give her a folded-up washcloth to see if the anger could move through her mouth. Debra bites down on it and shakes her head, muffling some loud sounds. With the anger now expressed and witnessed, Debra reaches for the young girl, lowers the bars, and takes her out of the hospital. The five-year-old sits on her lap. She holds the girl and tells her she is healthy now and can stay in the present with her. Debra's jaw feels much looser. Along with less jaw tension, it is easier for Debra to speak for her emotions and her needs.

Moving Forward with Grief and Loss

Lack of movement can be just as revealing. Jack sat across from me with his face, neck, and shoulders held stiffly. His partner had died a couple years ago, and his body expressed the paralyzing grief.

Jack: People keep telling me I should "move on" and get on with my life. They even are trying to set me up with other men. I may never be ready to do that. There will never be another Kyle for me. I'm not happy alone, but moving on feels impossible. It feels disloyal somehow. I still miss him. I've grieved and cried a lot, and maybe people are right. Maybe you can help me find a way to move on.

SM: I understand that the idea of moving on from the life you shared for thirty years with Kyle feels impossible and wrong to some part, and another part thinks you should. Can we find out more about this? Let's find a place in the room to represent the life you shared with Kyle. See how it feels to try to take a step away from this life.

Jack stands in the middle of the room and does not move.

Jack: Yeah. I just feel kinda stuck. I guess I just can't accept he is really gone.

With that, Jack returns to his seat, holds his head in his hands, and cries.

SM: Yes. Take some time to feel all those parts in your body that don't want you to move on. [*After some minutes, I continue.*] I wonder if there is another way to move, like to move with your grief, to move forward rather than to move on. Right now, can you find something in the room that represents the years you had with Kyle, the life you shared?

Jack: I have a photo with me of both of us.

Jack stands up, takes the photo out of his wallet, shows it to me, and holds it in his hand.

SM: OK. Now can you find something in the room that can stand for something you are moving toward in the future, even if it is something that seems small or insignificant?

Jack: Well . . . I have plans to go to the opera with some friends. I don't really want to go because it will make me feel sad, remembering how much Kyle loved the opera. I can have this bookcase be the opera.

SM: Good. Holding the photo, take a step toward the bookcase, representing going to the opera and taking your sadness, your grief, and your memories of your life with Kyle with you.

Jack holds the photo to his heart and takes a step toward the bookcase. He pauses, and then, with tears flowing, he takes another step.

Jack: I like the idea of "moving forward" rather than "moving on." I might be able to do that.

Conclusion

Metaphorically and literally, Mindful Movement can assist the process of Somatic IFS. Drawing upon the practices of awareness, breath, and resonance, we have established our relationship with the vertical plane and are moving from our heart into the horizontal plane. We bring mindful awareness to movements gross and subtle, habitual and interrupted, conscious and unconscious. We notice the rhythms, gestures, postures, and gait. We discover parts whose stories may best be told through these movements. The stories of interrupted motor development from conception through childhood are waiting for someone to listen. Inviting and welcoming the movements allows the stories held in the tissues to unfold.

We bring mindful awareness to the movements of yield, push, reach, grasp, and pull. As we yield, we feel the floor support us, even rise up to meet our body. As we yield even more, as our tension melts away and our body surrenders into this support below, from deep within our body eventually arises a delicious impulse to move, to feel our power, to push against, to push away. That movement leads to others. We may roll on the floor to allow every part of our body to also know the floor. Our limbs may want to rise up, to reach into space. Movement, large and small, fast and slow, free and choreographed, is a natural way for living beings to express their truest natures and their relationship to the grand wider world.

There are many bodymind movement practices that cultivate Embodied Self, such as various forms of yoga, Somatics, Feldenkrais, Alexander Technique, dance, and martial arts. Bringing awareness to parts that arise in the midst of practicing these movements, we can follow trailheads to the origins of the faulty movement patterns to correct them at the core rather than through repetition of a guided movement pattern.

We can also simply attend to the naturally occurring movements in our body. The movement of opening leads to the impulse to close. Extension eventually calls forth the action of flexion. Reaching out leads to the desire to rest, echoing the rhythmic cycles of nature. Tuning in to these cycles, lulled by the faint drumbeats of our internal rhythms, invigorated by the expression of our movement impulses, we express our Embodied Selves in movement.

When the emotional expression of a part is suppressed like a dampened fire, as with Jason's blocked impulse to hit, mindful awareness can ignite those embers and allow the blocked movement story to flow to completion. Initiating the appropriate developmental movements in a mindful state can act like tinder to a tiny spark of awareness, even with movements in utero, as with Thea, assisting clients to heal their relational traumas and develop secure attachment with their Embodied Self. Restoring and enacting mindfully the developmental movements, as in the session with Maya, can lead to a relational repair. Mindful Movement can resolve polarizations, as with Lori's push-pull of her eating disorder. When trauma and the resultant chronic pain freezes the body story in the past, as with Debra's jaw tension and Jack's locked-in grief, Mindful Movement allows the stories of trauma to emerge and the internal system to transform.

The practice of Mindful Movement can contact the preverbal matrix of the parts' experience directly. It can uncover the dormant impulses to move, allowing the frozen impulse and the emotions to sequence through the body. As the early movement patterns are reenacted, the associated memories and emotions may be accessed, allowing for witnessing and unburdening of the parts. The parts' burdens—acquired, inherited, or energetically transmitted intergenerationally—can be cleared through movement witnessed by Embodied Self. As the flow of the life force is restored, Embodied Self is expressed in powerful, graceful, integrated movement.

The exercises that follow can help the Somatic IFS therapist bring mindful awareness to their movements as a path to revealing and unburdening their parts. As our thoughts and emotions are accompanied by a muscular response, those responses become fixated in our movements. Largely outside our awareness, these movements tend to announce and reinforce our burdens. By exploring our habitual movements of posture, gait, and gestures we access a somatic record of our parts' burdened beliefs, emotions, and thoughts. Through movement the parts can be witnessed and their burdens released. Other exercises offer the opportunity to incrementally move through the developmental stages to access and witness implicitly held memories, to correct disturbances in the developing bodymind, and to reconnect us with our embryological wisdom and creativity. We can increase our capacity to hold our clients' relational traumas by reconnecting with our primal attachment experience and later developmental movements through our limbs, which become the template of our inner bodymind systems. As these exercises move us along the continuum of Embodied Self energy, possibilities for incorporating this practice of Mindful Movement into our therapeutic work will happen naturally.

EXERCISES

Mindfulness of Habitual Movements

PURPOSE   To bring curiosity to habitual movements and mindfully repeat them; to reveal those burdens embedded in our movement habits; to offer our parts the opportunity to be witnessed and their burdens released as they move through the body.

INSTRUCTIONS:

1. Select one habitual movement you want to explore. It could be a gesture you frequently make with your arms or hands, or a particular way you sit or stand, or something characteristic about the way you walk. You might want to ask a friend for their observation, or have someone record a video while you're walking, talking, or doing a daily activity. You could imagine being in a challenging situation to observe how your body automatically moves in reaction to it. You might bring mindfulness to the act of walking through a door, crossing the threshold into new territory, or coming upon a closed door. If you aren't sure what to focus on, just begin to move and allow your body to show you a focus for this exercise.

2. Notice how you feel toward this movement, and address any criticism or shame from a part until the part is willing to allow your full curiosity toward the movement.

3. Mindfully repeat the movement, being open to any thoughts, words, images, or emotions that seem to be connected with the movement.

4. If this leads you to a part, let the part feel your presence.

5. You can experiment with making the movement larger or smaller, faster or slower. You can allow the movement to take over your entire body, or be limited to a finger.

6. If it becomes clear that the part is a protector, you could try not doing the movement or changing the movement to find out

about the part's fears or who it is protecting. If the part holds some hurt, you could invite the part to show you its story of hurt through movement. Ask the part if there are other movements it wants to make, and invite the part to allow the story to move all the way through the body.

7. Find out if there are parts that don't want the story to flow.

8. Invite the part to tell the story with words or images.

REFLECTIONS:

1. What habitual movement did you explore? How did you initially feel toward it?

2. What happened when you repeated the movement mindfully?

3. Were there parts that resisted this exercise?

4. Was there a part using this movement to tell its story or do its job?

5. Were there any emotions, thoughts, or images connected with the movement?

6. Was the movement able to be released through the body?

7. When you repeat the movement now, is there any difference?

Yield, Push, and Reach through the Vertical Axis

PURPOSE To establish greater awareness of the core of the body, specifically the area of the navel, and the vertical axis of the body.

INSTRUCTIONS:

Allow yourself all the time you need, and frequently come back to *yield* to integrate the movements. If you feel any physical or emotional block or resistance as you perform a movement, mindfully explore it until you feel more ease and flow with the movement or until you find the part within the difficulty with the movement.

1. The first movement is *yield*. Lie on a mat or a rug on your back, knees bent. Invite your body to rest down onto the floor. Notice

the places on your body that touch the floor, and the places that don't. Take several breaths, allowing any unneeded muscle tension to dissolve with each exhale. Let the floor support you. Imagine it is rising up to meet you. Notice the difference between *yield* and *collapse*. Notice any parts in your body that are not yet ready to yield.

2. Bring awareness to your navel, your original place of connection. Place your hand on your navel; feel it rise and fall with your breath. Imagine a line from this center of your body to the center of the earth, a conduit through which you can receive from and release into the earth.

3. On an exhale press your lumbar area into the floor so it makes contact with the floor. This is the movement of *push*. Do this a few times, alternating between the movements of yield and push.

4. Alternate the movements of push and yield from your navel to your tail, and then from your navel to your head, all along your vertebrae.

5. Staying connected with the earth from your navel, *reach* upward with your tailbone, then yield; reach with the top of your head, then yield. Reach with your eyes, nose, mouth, tongue, then yield. Reach in any direction with your tail, and with your head, then yield.

6. Roll onto each of your sides and your stomach and continue to explore yielding, pushing, and reaching through your head and tail. Flex and extend along this vertical axis, from navel to tail, and from navel to head. These movements connect the organs, glands, and other body structures and energy centers of the body.

7. Continue exploring these movements from head to tail on all fours, then sitting, then standing.

REFLECTIONS:

1. What was your experience when connecting through your navel to the earth?

2. You practiced the movements of yield, push, and reach from your navel to your head and to your tail. How did each one feel? Which ones were easy, satisfying, even joyful? What qualities of Self energy did you find in these movements?

3. What/who were you yielding to? What/who were you pushing against? What/who were you reaching for?

4. Were there any blocks along the line from navel to tip of limb? Which ones presented a challenge—a resistance, a weakness, a disconnection, confusion or irritation? Did any feelings, thoughts, words, or images arise as you did these movements?

5. Was there a difference lying on your back, sides, or stomach?

6. As you moved your vertical axis, from head to tail, were there any places along this axis where you found a part wanting attention?

7. Was there a way these movements were restorative for you?

Yield, Push, and Reach through the Six Limbs of the Body

PURPOSE To mindfully revisit early expressions of the embryo's agency via the four limbs.

INSTRUCTIONS:

Allow yourself all the time you need, and frequently come back to *yield* to integrate the movements. If you feel any physical or emotional block or resistance as you perform a movement, mindfully explore it until you feel more ease and flow with the movement or until you find the part within the difficulty with the movement. Listen to your body's movement impulses rather than strictly following the instructions.

1. Lie on your back and reconnect with your navel and the movement of *yield*.

2. Starting with one arm, bring awareness to each of your four limbs and the line from the middle of your body at your navel all the way down to your fingertips and your toes.

3. Invite each limb to yield to the floor below.

4. Experiment with the movement *push* from this central core to a limb, one limb at a time, noticing any differences between the experience with each limb.

5. Explore this push movement with more than one limb: both arms, both legs, limbs on the right side, limbs on the left side, all together, and finally diagonally, each time moving between push and yield as you listen to the impulse from your body. Consider exploring these movements as you change your position to lying on your side or stomach, or sitting or standing.

6. The next movement you can explore through your four limbs is *reach*. When you feel the impulse to reach, reach with your arm from your central core to your fingertips. You might want to eventually experiment with reaching with both arms, both legs, right side, left side, all four limbs simultaneously.

7. Continue to play with these three movements through your six limbs, lying on the floor, on all fours, sitting, standing. See how these movements take you through space.

REFLECTIONS:

1. Draw how your body feels after having explored these movements of yield, push, and reach through each of your four limbs.

2. What/who were you yielding to? What/who were you pushing against? What/who were you reaching for?

3. How did each of the three movements feel through each of your limbs? Which ones were easy, satisfying, even joyful? What qualities of Self energy did you find in these movements?

4. Were there any blocks along the line from navel to tip of limb? Which ones presented a challenge—a resistance, a weakness, a disconnection, confusion or irritation? Did any feelings, thoughts, words, or images arise as you did these movements?

5. Make a note of what you noticed in order to revisit the movement and spend more time with the parts associated with the movement, to restore a disrupted movement, or to enjoy a restorative movement experience.

6

Attuned Touch: Exploring the
Power of Ethical Touch

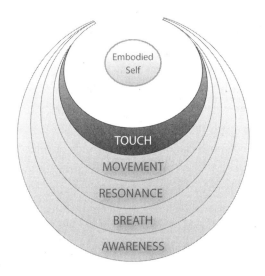

IN THE SOMATIC IFS logo this final practice of Attuned Touch appears
as if it is being hugged by the four practices that lie below it. The practices of
awareness, breath, resonance, and movement provide the foundation and
container for touch to join them as a channel of implicit communication

between parts and Self. The image portrays that the embracing successive support of each of the underlying practices ensures that this powerful practice will be attuned, appropriate, and ethical.

Somatic Awareness is important for both the one being touched and the one doing the touching. Awareness of our body lets us know when we want touch, what kind of touch, and what happens when we are touched. Of all the senses, touch is the only one that is reciprocal. We cannot touch another without being touched ourselves.[1] Interoception is essential for both parties, as is the therapist's exteroception as they track the client's somatic responses to the touch. Conscious Breathing calms the nervous system to be able to accept and receive touch. The act of breathing touches us internally. Breath opens the space for a resonant relationship. Compassion flows from an open heart through to the hand. Receptivity and revision, aspects of Radical Resonance, take concrete form in this practice, deepening the connection and participating in this intimate, implicit flesh-to-flesh communication. Attuned Touch is nestled in the embrace of Mindful Movement. The impulse to touch may begin with a movement as a hand spontaneously touches the place in the body that is asking for contact. Subtle movements in the tissues being touched may reveal the part's implicit story as well as its resolution.

The uppermost position of Attuned Touch implies reliance on the underlying practices to ensure that touch interventions will be from Embodied Self rather than from a part. Its proximity to Embodied Self infers that, in some cases, touch may be the most direct and effective means for a part to sense the presence of Self energy. Even more than tone of voice, facial expression, or posture, touch tacitly conveys the therapist's inner state in the relationship. My experience as a bodyworker has familiarized me with numerous well-meaning parts whose energy, I assume, is being readily transmitted from flesh to flesh. Parts looking for what is wrong, parts needing to make right in order to feel valued, insecure and inadequate parts, timid parts, overconfident parts. The qualities of Self energy are communicated as well. Whether the touch is from the therapist, from the client, or if the touch is imagined in the client's inner scenario, touch offers an additional and often more effective nonverbal route for a

Self-to-part relationship. The Self energy transmitted through touch travels in a continual feedback loop supported by the sensorimotor system.

In addition to being sequential, all the practices of Somatic IFS are interdependent and reciprocal. Attuned Touch weaves throughout all of them in a unique way. Touch is initially contingent on awareness, and touch can awaken and heighten awareness. Touch can focus our attention on a part in our body when our mind wants to drift away and jump around. Placing our hands on the places that move as we breathe, we are more conscious of our breathing. Our touch can ease restrictions. Just as healing touch relies on an attuned relationship, the stream of biochemicals released from the touch reinforces and expedites a safe, healing, resonant relationship. While movement initiates touch, bringing touch to a stuck or frozen place in the body frees up the movement that can restore the flow of energy in the bodymind system.

Attuned Touch as seen in the graphic is also the smallest of all the practices. This suggests that the amount of time using touch in a typical Somatic IFS session is less than the other practices. Touch is intimate. A little can go a long way, and often even brief physical contact can evoke a strong response. Touch from the therapist may not be appropriate for some clients, or for all clients at some times. Touch is filled with many layers of meaning, both psychological and cultural. The sexual, touch, and trauma history of the client and therapist, the culture and religion of the client and therapist, and the gendered or hierarchical nature of the therapist–client relationship are just some of the layers. The evoked meanings of touch are often outside of the client's conscious awareness, and even more often are not articulated, yet they will manifest in the body and in the relationship. The Somatic IFS practices underlying Attuned Touch offer the tools for assessing appropriate safe boundaries around this powerful practice and for reading and responding to the messages from touch.

The relatively small size of this practice also reflects the influence of a culture that fears and avoids touch. Western culture conflates touch with sex, power, and dominance and sexualizes or infantilizes the meaning of touch. Therapists who fear their touch will be misinterpreted avoid any kind of touch, especially in the US with its litigious culture, and the field of psychotherapy has mostly taken a "hands-off" stance. Touch in psychotherapy, and in our culture in general, is fraught with controversy, constrained by professional regulations based on fear-based risk management practices. Although well-intentioned, these cultural protective parts leave clients deprived of the touch that could heal their touch wounds.

There are many national, regional, ethnic, and racial differences regarding touch practices. In the US, whites touch less than people of color. Developmental psychologist Sharon Heller tells us that American infants and children are touched less than in most other countries, which she attributes in part to an overreliance on infant carriers, strollers, swings, pacifiers, bottles, and cribs.[2] Another study shows that harsh and punitive touch outweighs the affectionate touch in American child-rearing practices.[3] There is a classic touch study known as the "coffee shop study," conducted in the 1960s by Canadian psychologist Sidney Jourard, that has often been interpreted to demonstrate intercultural differences in touch.[4] While sitting in cafés in several countries, he counted the number of times pairs of people touched each other in an hour. Not surprisingly, people in London and the US touched nearly not at all, while in France and Puerto Rico they hardly kept their hands off each other. The idea of replicating his study with a more thorough and systematic methodology has a certain appeal.

My anecdotal evidence of cultural differences regarding touch comes from my experiences teaching internationally. When I have taught in France, Germany, Spain, and Portugal we all greet each other every morning with warm hugs and a kiss on both cheeks, and we bid goodbye each evening in the same way. In the US, UK, and Japan, there is a sense of restraint with touching among us all. As familiarity and trust develops, hugs increase. Many participants in the UK training said they had no memory of being touched by their parents except for punishment, and for those who attended British boarding schools there were strict rules against any kind of physical contact between the students. As I sit in airports waiting to be flown to these countries, I observe touch and lack of it. I see children in their strollers glued to iPads while parents gaze at their cell phones.

The cultural taboo against touch in psychotherapy encourages therapists to perpetuate the neglect that originally caused the injury. Because of the immense potential of touch to heal and to harm, this overlooked communication pathway from a part to Embodied Self, and to the part from Embodied Self, is used judiciously and wisely in Somatic IFS, with permission of all the parts.

I have to admit that even in my trainings I don't give this practice the time it deserves. Regardless of the length of the training, I tend to borrow a little time from touch for the other practices, feeling that each deserves and, indeed, requires a lifetime to adequately master, and then I squeeze Attuned Touch into the remaining time. And yet I claim the most mastery in the practice of touch, having studied and practiced various forms of bodywork for over thirty years. I have experienced the power of touch in healing wounds of body and mind for myself and countless clients. The neglect of this practice cannot simply be attributed to flawed time management. My parts have absorbed these cultural beliefs, and they believe that by minimizing the place of touch in the compendium of practices I can avoid stirring up controversy.

Contrary to my parts' fears, however, it is the practice of Attuned Touch that has lately been drawing the most attention of all the Somatic IFS practices. Participants in my trainings have asked for further training in the use of touch. Some have suggested that just as IFS is on the cutting edge of psychotherapy, Somatic IFS is on the cutting edge of IFS, and Attuned Touch is on the cutting edge of Somatic IFS. During my professional life numerous research studies have shown touch to be a vital component of healing in a wide range of clinical issues. The current, more open climate in psychotherapy ushers in the potential for appropriate, ethical, skillful touch to take a more prominent role in healing today than it has in the past. All of this is helping me regard this practice as the jewel on the crown of Somatic IFS practices. The complexity and the potential of touch for healing bodies and cultures demands that this practice receive its deserved attention. Perhaps as touch is recognized and practiced in psychotherapy it will become the bridge that joins the two artificially disparate fields of body and mind.

If it can be said that some psychotherapists are too cautious about touch, perhaps bodyworkers and other healthcare professionals are not cautious enough. In many cases they are not sufficiently aware that their touch may stir up trauma and other unresolved issues lying dormant in the tissues of their clients' bodies. I have heard healthcare professionals claim they have had no clients or patients with a history of trauma. Many dentists, nurses, doctors, physical therapists, and other practitioners involved in diagnostic and treatment procedures involving touch don't ask for permission or feedback. Most bodyworkers and massage therapists invite the client to give them feedback about the touch and to let them know if they want anything different. However, even when invited, when I am lying on a table naked under a thin sheet as the bodyworker is busily executing their protocol, I find it difficult to speak up. I know of several instances where deep and invasive touch has resulted in harm to the client. In addition to the power to heal, touch has the power to harm both the relationship and, ultimately, the client. Bodywork training provides the practitioner with expertise in their particular method but can't fully attend to the minefield of psychological complexities of the touch histories within the bodies lying on their tables. To help meet this need, I developed, along with Hakomi trainer Morgan Holford, a training for bodyworkers to help them work safely and ethically within the bounds of their profession with the emotions that are embedded in the tissues, fluids, and organs.

My visual teaching materials for Attuned Touch include Michelangelo's creation scene in the Sistine Chapel that portrays God's gift of life bestowed upon Adam as they reach toward each other through their outstretched arms. Yet when we look closely, we see their fingers don't actually touch. As our eyes are drawn to this space between their delicately depicted index fingers, we experience the chasm in our relationship with the divine. We sense our own longing to connect in an embodied way with the world of Spirit. Although spiritual relationships are often conceptualized as disembodied experiences, people of all faiths are moved by Michelangelo's portrayal of the magical potential of touch to open the door to a deeper connection with Spirit.

This practice portrayed at the apex of the practices of Somatic IFS returns us to our roots. Touch is our first language, both chronologically and psychologically. Anthropologist and educator Ashley Montagu's seminal work *Touching: The Human Significance of the Skin*[5] brings together studies demonstrating the major role of touch in human development. He tells us that touch is the first sensory system to develop in animals, and that all of our other senses are derived from it. Touch as a primary means of connection begins in the womb. Within three weeks of conception, we have developed a primitive nervous system that links skin cells to our rudimentary brain. At about eight weeks after conception, the sense of touch develops. Long before we can see, hear, smell, or taste, through our sense of touch we begin to receive and process information about ourselves and our outer world. Bonnie Bainbridge Cohen of Body-Mind Centering tells us movement and touch develop at the same time in utero, and they both nourish us throughout our life, within and without. She describes the embryo swimming in the amniotic ocean, constantly bumping up against the uterine wall. Through this skin-to-skin contact the embryo comes to know the difference between the world inside and outside their skin, which becomes the basis for differentiation and individuation.[6]

After birth, touch continues to be the primary language of the infant. The warm, sensual, physical contact between infant and caregiver establishes a bonding even more crucial than food for healthy development. Touch is a building block of secure attachment. When the touch is attuned to the infant, communicating security, safety, and belonging, the infant develops the secure attachment that becomes the foundation for their later relational lives. Not enough touch, or the wrong kind of touch, results in developmental trauma and lifelong adverse ramifications. For parts with wounds of attachment, as with our clients' infant or pre-birth parts, touch can be the most effective communication. Tactile experiences remain central to our emotions, our thought processes, and our healing throughout our life.

Many of our clients have not had enough of the right kind and too much of the wrong kind of touch. They have absorbed many psychological and physiological burdens that affect their personal lives. They may be over- or under-responsive to touch. They may reject and resist touch or may lack the ability to set touch boundaries. They may have parts that yearn for touch or parts that seek inappropriate touch. Wounds of touch can be healed by reparative touch. When the client as a child experienced touch neglect, touch from the therapist and/or the client or imaginary touch can begin the process of relational repair of the client's bodymind attachment system. When the client can open to touch that carries the implicit message of safety and connection, of comfort and pleasure, their young parts can now receive the touch that is necessary for their secure attachment with the adult Self.

Barbara had a skin rash on her arms that had not responded to medical treatments. When she gently touched the rash to tune in to it and ask it what it was telling her, she heard a part say her skin was the place where she met the world, and the world was not safe. Barbara then got an image of a baby longing for touch. The rash told her she was protecting the baby from the longing, fearing the inevitable disappointment would again pull her into a vacuum of terrifying nothingness. Barbara gently stroked her arms, giving the baby the tactile attention she had longed for. The rash on her arm soon resolved but later showed up in other areas of her body. It turned out the rash was the first sign of some deeper emotions connected with both abandonment and trauma arising to the surface of her body.

Attuned Touch, like all the practices of Somatic IFS, can assist with every step of IFS. Attuned Touch addresses all the various coalitions of parts in the inner system, including the parts polarized about touch. Whether the touch is from the client or the therapist, or simply imagined, the oxytocin released from touch can deepen the bond between the parts and the Self. Touch can reveal a part in the body and help keep the attention focused on that part. Touch may serve to calm the nervous system and help the client unblend from emotionally dysregulated parts. Soft strokes to the arms or back speak directly to the insula and other limbic structures to calm them and communicate safety and emotional support. The client's or the therapist's touch can "listen" to the part's body story. The touch may perceive the tissues tighten, shake, and tremble, or soften and melt. The hands may pick up the energy of dissociation or disconnection. Touch can facilitate the unfolding movement story by assisting with the curling up, providing a hand to push away from, or firmly touching the feet to the ground to help the client orient to the present. Words, images, or feelings from the part may fill out the body story. The client, in charge of the kind of touch and the amount of touch, has a reparative experience. The client's parts can let go of past meanings and associations of touch violations and replace them with associations of comfort, connection, and pleasure.

Touch is often the most potent form of implicit communication between parts and Self. *New Yorker* writer Adam Gopnik writes about a specific research study on affective touch that was conducted by Dacher Keltner, a professor of psychology at the University of California Berkeley.[7] (As a specialist in the science of emotions, Keltner was the scientific advisor on Pixar's *Inside Out*.) Keltner's study involved 212 volunteers identifying twelve different emotions, one at a time, conveyed through a one-second touch to a stranger's forearm when both parties were separated by a barrier; the person being touched had to guess the emotion. Given the number of emotions tested, the odds of guessing the correct emotion connected with the touch were 8 percent. With emotions of compassion, gratitude, anger, love, and fear, the participants guessed correctly over half the time. They did much better identifying emotions from this touch than from visual or auditory cues.

Listening and Speaking with Our Hands

When psychotherapists tell me they feel they need more training in touch techniques in order to be comfortable using touch with their clients, I respond that being in a state of Embodied Self energy trumps any techniques. Attuned Touch can be enhanced by training in various forms of bodywork or Reiki or other hands-on or energetic method, but it does not require them. When our burdened parts are not taking over our hands, communicating and healing with our hands is our natural state. Listening with our hands is just as natural to us as listening with our ears. And just as we can train our ears to better distinguish sounds in our environment, we can also train our hands to hear the subtle, implicit language of the body. And we can guide our clients to listen and speak to their parts with their hands as well.

It was through working with clay that I first learned to listen with my hands. Kneading it, then softening it with water, my hands learned to sense what form this clay body was wanting to become. Pressing down, pulling up, opening up the top of the spinning ball, I felt the shape emerge and evolve. The round, full space inside the pot and the outside shape spoke to my hands about the kind of touch and when it had enough. Too much touch and it would weaken and collapse. Too little and it would look heavy and uninteresting.

My first bodywork teacher helped me translate this knowledge into touching bodies. Rather than prescribing a protocol of techniques, she coached me to simply listen to what the tissues under my hands were wanting, and to track the moment-by-moment changes. Shedding my ideas, fears, and insecurities, I was left with a willingness to connect, to send and receive. I simply placed my hands on the body before me. I sent openness and curiosity. I received messages of tightness, resistance, deadness, weakness, and fragility. My hands communicated acceptance and, in response, noticed movement, melting, softening, and opening.

My later extensive study of anatomy enhanced my listening and seeing through my hands. I became more acquainted with the muscles and fascia, the viscera and fluid systems. Visualizing the interiority of the body accompanied and augmented the sensory experience. Other bodywork trainings helped develop what Aline LaPierre has called "palpatory literacy."[8] Although specific touch training is valuable, my advice to psychotherapists who fear they don't have enough training in touch is the same given to me by my first bodywork teacher: "Trust your hands." And now I add "Separate from your parts." My advice to bodyworkers and health practitioners is the same—to hold their techniques, assumptions, protocols, and agendas to the side and tune in to the client or patient.

I learned this lesson many years ago from my bodywork client Paula. Paula was a survivor of sexual abuse and was referred to me by her psychotherapist. She had gone through the ten sessions of a traditional Rolfing treatment, which she said she benefitted from, and which I knew to be a type of bodywork that could engender intense responses both physically and emotionally. From this information I made some incorrect assumptions about her level of body awareness, but my body and her tissues told me otherwise. I felt disconnected from her, and I did not sense her fascia responding to my touch.

I stopped the bodywork and asked Paula to tell me in more detail about her experience being Rolfed. The story emerged of her staggering out of her first session onto the busy street and somehow finding a pay phone (yes, this was many years ago!) to call a friend to pick her up. She made it through the remaining nine sessions of Rolfing the same way she made it through the sexual abuse, by dissociating from her body. Her protectors were making sure she did not again get overwhelmed by her memories of her abuse. We worked together to find how she could receive touch without leaving her body. I guided her to begin by bringing awareness to the sensations in the tip of one small finger for five seconds. She gradually included her hand, arm, and eventually the rest of her body. Starting with her own touch and then cautiously including mine, she came to tolerate the touch as long as she could control it. Eventually she was able to notice the kind of touch she liked and the kind she didn't. It turned out she was exceptionally aware and discriminating. She found she could ask me for the kind of touch that helped her enjoy the pleasurable sensations. Paula told me she "got her body back."

Our hands also have the ability to speak. Energetically we connect with our heart and send warmth and presence through our hands to the parts inhabiting the tissues. We can also send words, spoken or unspoken, such as "I am here," "I'm listening," "I hear you," "It's OK now." We can gently inquire, "What are you wanting me to know?" "What are you afraid of?" "Are you ready to let that go?" We verbally speak as well, asking how parts are responding to the touch, if this is exactly the kind of touch they are wanting, what they might want to try instead. Especially with clients with known sexual touch violations, it is important to explicitly state that the touch will not be sexual and that they are completely in charge of the touch. We are listening and speaking with all of our senses as we track the internal bodymind system.

Body System Associated with Attuned Touch

The Somatosensory System

The skin is the visible part of this somatosensory system, which is also referred to as the tactile system. The skin is the interface between "me" and "not me." Our sense of our identity, including our beauty, is, to a large degree, skin deep. Our skin is the boundary between everything inside us and everything outside us, guarding against foreign invasion and excessive fluid loss. Yet it is more than a neutral envelope. This boundary gets pierced, sometimes with our permission, sometimes by accident, sometimes for healing, sometimes for wounding. It is through this membrane and the neural structures linked to it that we feel into the outside world. Through our skin we learn what to avoid, what to move toward, what to embrace. Our skin teaches us about ourselves. We learn to be comfortable in our own skin, or not.

The skin is our body's largest, oldest, and most sensitive organ. It is the most active source of sensations in the body. In an average-size man the skin weighs about nine pounds and takes up about eighteen square feet. Below the level of awareness the skin is handling metabolic activities, temperature regulation, healing, immunity, and excretion. But the function most critical to our survival and our overall physical and mental health is the skin's sensory activities.

Deane Juhan in his book *Job's Body* refers to the skin as the outer layer of the brain.[9] There are many associations between the skin and the brain, beginning in the first days after conception where the cells are forming three primitive layers along a vertical axis. The somatosensory system developed from the back layer of cells, referred to as the ectoderm, that originally formed the protective structures of the amniotic sac. This fluid-filled sac offered vital protection to our earliest formation. As our embryo developed rapidly, its structures formed and re-formed in overlapping waves arising out of this embryonic cell layer. Within three weeks after our conception, our ectoderm develops a primitive nervous system, linking our skin cells to our rudimentary brain. From this primitive structure of the amniotic sac through the many transformations of our ectoderm, our body serves the need for communication and protection. The structure of the amniotic sac has radically transformed, but the protective function remains, as skin and nervous system are linked through our somatosensory system to provide protection as well as relational communication throughout our life.

The burdens we carry from touch abuse and neglect are embedded in our somatosensory system. The burdens concern the ways in which the inherent protection and communication was inadequate to prevent harm. Our somatosensory system also holds the source of healing these wounds. The embodiment of our creativity and resiliency in our tactile system can be accessed through Attuned Touch.

Juhan describes the complex processes of the somatosensory system as the receiver and arbiter of touch. There are two pathways of this touch that operate simultaneously, the *afferent* pathway from skin to brain, and the *efferent* pathway from brain to skin. The parts of this system involved in the afferent flow of signals—the skin and the various sensory receptors and afferent neurons in the skin, muscles, and organs and the spinal cord, brain stem, thalamus, and the somatosensory cortex—receive information about the touch. Each type of receptor activates a different part of the brain, responding to the many kinds of touch—loving touch, sexual touch, violent touch, abusive touch, and healing touch. The somatosensory cortex encodes all this incoming sensory information and makes meaning of it.

The efferent pathway conducts impulses from the brain to the periphery. Thoughts and emotions affect the skin and the embedded neurons. Positive sensory experiences that are introduced—safe, soothing, connected, respectful touch—create new neural patterns, relaxing chronically tense or collapsed muscles. Juhan explains the process of healing touch:

> It must use tactile sensations to reach the mind, the whole mind, from the surface of the skin to the spinal reflexes, to the subconscious responses of the lower brain, to the fields of awareness of the cortex. When this happens, touch is genuinely, profoundly therapeutic.[10]

Tiffany Field's research gives us more information about how therapeutic touch specifically affects the somatosensory system.[11] From her studies we have learned that when skin is moved and touched it stimulates specific receptors for pressure that slow heart rate, reduce blood pressure, and release cortisol and neuropeptides. Touch unleashes a stream of healing chemical responses, including an increase in serotonin and dopamine and the number of killer cells in the immune system. Still other specialized touch receptors exist solely to communicate emotion and to form social bonds—which are coded completely differently from other sensory information, involving specialized peripheral nerve fibers that perceive a gentle caress. Interestingly, scientists have even determined the ideal speed of a human caress, which they tell us is three to five centimeters a second. The feeling of pleasure produced by this touch activates a different part of the brain, the anterior cingulate cortex, the area implicated in several cognitive functions such as empathy, emotions, impulse control, and decision making. This area is considered to be responsible for many aspects of our well-being throughout our life span.

Elements Associated with Attuned Touch

Having associated each of the four classical elements with the first four of the Somatic IFS practices, I wonder about this fifth practice. These four elements were considered by ancient cultures to be the basis of the material world. They were associated with deities and were used to explain physical bodies as well as mystical phenomena. Aristotle added a fifth element, ether, sometimes referred to as a void. But touch is anything but ethereal, nor is it meant to be a path to the abyss. I have solved the dilemma by deciding this practice incorporates them all.

Just as Attuned Touch relies on the underlying Somatic IFS practices, the four elements are united in the interplay of earth, air, water, and fire. The therapist connects with earth for grounding prior to physical contact. Making contact, the therapist engages in the sensory, earthy aspects of skin-to-skin contact. Tuning in to the surrounding space, the therapist accesses the element of air. This opens the therapist to their internal spaciousness and also to receiving information from the wider Field of Self energy that can inform the therapeutic touch. Water brings flow to tissues that resemble beef jerky and heart-felt compassion to seemingly impenetrable boundaries. The element of fire as a transformative agent is channeled in the soothing warmth of a hand to comfort and relax parts held in tense tissues. Each of the four elements or all of them together support the practice of Attuned Touch, and they link the healing practice of Somatic IFS with healing and spiritual practices throughout the ages.

Controversy Concerning Touch in Healing and Psychotherapy

The use of touch for healing is as ancient as the need for healing both mind and body. The earliest recorded medical histories show that touch was used for healing in Egypt and China. From at least 3000 BCE, healing touch was used in Ayurvedic medicine. The controversy concerning touch for healing is almost as old as the practice of healing touch itself. Beginning in the Middle Ages, lay touch healers were oppressed and stigmatized and finally exiled or burned at the stake; human touch was replaced by leeches sucking out the "humours."

The use of touch in psychotherapy echoes the cycle of acceptance and prohibition of touch. Sigmund Freud used touch in the early days to facilitate emotional expression and age regression in his patients, but unfortunately he conflated the infant's desire for touch with sexuality. His later focus on the role of transference caused him to abandon the use of touch, which his colleague Wilhelm Reich tried to remedy by using touch to liberate his patients from their body armor. Touch violations among the psychoanalytic community resulted in the pendulum swinging toward prohibition. Clashes between Freud and his colleagues over the place of touch in psychoanalysis, and associating all forms of touch with sexuality, foreshadowed our current controversies.

An article available from the Zur Institute describes how the pendulum swung back in favor of touch after WWII as research by John Bowlby and Mary Ainsworth led the psychological community to understand the connection between touch and attachment.[12] The Zur article describes how Harry Harlow "took Bowlby's theory to the lab" when he conducted a variety of experiments with rhesus macaque monkeys to assess the impact of maternal deprivation and the need for interactive touch to support normal development.

In my undergraduate studies I was introduced to the films of Harlow's classic work. My heart still aches when I recall viewing those infants separated from their mothers at birth and given a choice between a terry cloth–covered mesh structure and a bare wire structure fitted with bottles, and how they clung pathetically to the soft structure yet still became self-mutilating and asocial. It occurred to me that many human newborns don't get enough touch, as they are plopped into an isolated crib shortly after birth. Harlow's experiments left a lasting impact on my professional development, but more widely his research—along with the work of child analysts and researchers—was a step toward scientific legitimacy of the importance of tactile stimulation for healthy psychological development.

More recent research in the last half century has validated the importance of touch for human development, bonding, and communication, which has bolstered the consideration of touch as an appropriate psychotherapeutic intervention, especially with touch neglect. Ashley Montagu wrote poetically and yet convincingly: "When the need for touch remains unsatisfied, abnormal behavior will result."[13] The "abnormal behavior" associated with touch neglect has social as well as psychological consequences. James Prescott, a neuroscientist formerly with the US Department of Health, Education, and Welfare, reviewed forty-nine societies and concluded that the primary cause of violent behavior in adults is the lack of touching and stroking during the formative periods of their lives.[14] Many social researchers have concluded that American babies and children are among the least touched on Earth, and they have suggested a link with the high level of violence in the US compared to other developed countries that have a higher amount of touch.

Later research has demonstrated the significant benefits of touch in many other arenas, from preterm newborns' health to NBA basketball team performance, class participation, and even library attendance. Since the 1980s the research of Tiffany Field, through the Touch Research Institute at the University of Miami School of Medicine, has contributed enormously to the body of research regarding the efficacy of touch for physical and emotional healing of people of all ages. Field has demonstrated that touch lessens the physical symptoms that cannot be separated from emotional ones, such as pain, cortisol levels, blood glucose, and cardiac stress, and improves immunity and pulmonary function. Her book *Touch* includes results of these studies that cite the efficacy of touch for healing a wide range of clinical issues such as anxiety, depression, hyperactivity, attention deficits, grief, PTSD, addictions, and, of course, physical symptoms.

Appreciation of the necessity of touch clashes with recognition of the potential harm of touch amplified by media reports of sexual exploitation and inappropriate touch. Edward Smith opens his book *Touch in Psychotherapy* with the words "Shrouded for many in a cloak of fear, rumor and misinformation, touch is perhaps the most controversial topic in psychotherapy today."[15] Abuse perpetrated by therapists and institutions shadows the profession. History is rife with incidents that show the potential of touch for healing and harm in any profession with differential power dynamics.

Touch and trauma is even more controversial than other clinical issues. A high level of sensitivity is required to navigate this territory. So much trauma happens through physical contact: physical abuse, physical assault, combat, sexual abuse, serious accidents, even medical procedures. Parts of traumatized people desperately crave touch, while simultaneously other parts are terrified of body contact and won't allow the person to want it or receive it. Touch may cause traumatized parts to feel trapped, afraid, vulnerable, sexually stimulated, or numbed out. Touch can be overwhelmingly confusing because the trauma has damaged their ability to distinguish between safe and unsafe touch. Touch may be contraindicated with some trauma survivors until their system is healed enough to benefit from the healing power of touch described earlier.

Body therapist and author Babette Rothschild considers individual differences with regard to touch in healing trauma.[16] She cautions against touch by the therapist with "Type II B" clients (those who have experienced multiple traumas); she fears that the transference and countertransference could become intense and uncontainable. Instead she suggests that the therapist support the client to learn to ask for, receive, and utilize touch among their network of close family, friends, and in therapy group situations. While getting the touch, the client can track their heart and breathing rates and restore their ability to say yes and no to touch.

Bessel van der Kolk, one of the foremost therapists, researchers, and writers on the topic of healing trauma, strongly advocates the use of touch.[17] In *The Body Keeps the Score* he highlights touch as the most elementary tool for calming the system. He speaks compassionately of traumatized bodies and suggests that we quiet them down the same way that we quiet down babies—by holding, touching, and rocking them, being in tune with them, and very gradually exposing them to new things. He encourages all his patients to engage in some kind of bodywork.

Over the last couple decades, countless research studies have pointed to the healing potential of touch for traumatized clients and indicated that the physiological and emotional effects of trauma can be reversed through touch. Brain research has shown that touch causes the hypothalamus to release oxytocin, and it can spur the prefrontal cortex to grow GABA-bearing fibers down to the amygdala and quell the fear response. Tiffany Field's research with traumatized people shows that touch helps with many symptoms such as aversion to touch, distorted body image, anxiety, depression, high cortisol levels, and high blood pressure. Touch repairs traumatized clients' self-esteem, trust, and a sense of their own power or agency, especially in setting limits and asking for what they need. According to polyvagal theory, touch can activate the ventral vagus and assist with emotional regulation. The first impulse in the face of a threat is to reach out, and that impulse is overridden by the more primitive ANS responses that kick into gear. Touch can restore the ventral vagal nerve's social-engagement impulse to reach out, as well as other impulses that have been exiled.

The abundant research and writing concerning the necessity and efficacy of touch has supported the emergence of many body-oriented therapies that utilize touch, such as Bioenergetics, Adlerian and Gestalt therapy, Hakomi, Somatic Experiencing, and Sensorimotor Psychotherapy, and even Satir's family therapy as well as some cognitive and behavioral approaches. Somatic IFS has been influenced and nourished by many of these approaches.

Yet despite all the evidence of touch's potential to repair wounds of attachment and the effect of touch abuses—emotionally, somatically, socially, even neurologically—the fears and confusions are deeply embedded in the field, causing many psychotherapists to still regard touch as dangerous, inappropriate, unethical, or irrelevant in their clinical work. They fear evoking romantic, sexual, or perpetrator transferential relationships. Although these fears deserve to be validated, they can rob the profession of reparative interventions in clinical and educational work with individuals, couples, and families. The taboo against touching reflects and exacerbates disconnection and dissociation from the body. It is important to consider that withholding touch as a therapeutic intervention with clients who missed out on necessary touch may further the wound of touch neglect.

The controversies about the use of touch attest to the power of touch to both harm and heal. The intention to safeguard both clients and therapists from the consequences of unethical touch with strict regulations and prohibitions unfortunately has not prevented touch abuses. Research shows it is therapists' burdens around touch that are the risk for touch abuses. These parts need healing, not to be shamed, frightened, and controlled by risk management approaches, ethical review boards, and insurance companies. The best insurance against touch violations is for us practitioners to resolve our own wounds of touch neglect or abuse. This work is essential for therapists practicing Attuned Touch.

Training and supervision in the appropriate, ethical use of touch is also crucial. The Zur Institute offers online continuing education courses for mental health practitioners in the ethical use of touch. Body psychotherapist and author Courtenay Young calls for clearer ethical guidelines for appropriate touch, including bringing awareness to the therapeutic impact of handshakes, hugs, kisses on the cheek, or pats on the back. The United States Association for Body Psychotherapy (USABP) publishes their code of ethics online, and the section "Ethics of Touch" is included at the end of this chapter. While appreciating the importance of touch, Young, a leader in the field of body psychotherapy, understands equally the need for guidelines to determine when touch is and is not appropriate or ethical:

> There are also . . . many situations where it is clinically or psychotherapeutically inappropriate to touch, and doing so might be seen as counterproductive, crossing appropriate boundaries, or even being abusive. There are also situations where it may be inappropriate not to touch, and doing so could be seen as being cold, remote, distant, inaccessible, unfeeling, or contraindicative to the person's psychotherapeutic process.[18]

Attuned Touch in Somatic IFS

The practice of Attuned Touch takes in both of Young's considerations and attempts to alleviate the controversy and remove the touch taboo. In the teaching segment on the practice of Attuned Touch, there are several ways we work to ensure appropriate and ethical touch. The practices of awareness, breathing, and resonance provide a foundation for the toucher (either the client or the therapist) to be in a state of Embodied Self. In this state of connection to their body and supported by the wider Self Field, and in a resonant connection with the person being touched, the toucher can track the responses—before and during the touching episode—for nonverbal reactions to the touch within their own body and the body of the person being touched.

Participants in trainings explore their touch histories and the influence of our particular cultural norms regarding touch to find parts carrying burdens from harmful and deficient touch. Most all of us hold these wounds, and these burdens will interfere with our Embodied Self–led touch. Young parts deprived of touch may look to get soothed by cuddling with clients. Parts harmed by touch may fear and avoid touch or feel inadequate. Parts confused about appropriate professional boundaries might be tempted to act on their sexual attractions. Caretaking protectors might want to demonstrate their touch proficiency. Even if our touch falls within current ethical guidelines, parts' burdens will likely be conveyed through the touch, very possibly causing harm.

The practice of Attuned Touch harnesses the healing potential of this intervention while avoiding harmful touch—not only sexual touch but subtler forms of touch from the therapist's parts, such as parts needing the physical contact for soothing their own discomfort. Aware of the client's burdened parts and of their stage in their healing process, the therapist considers if touch is appropriate. Resolving their own burdens around touch, being grounded and supported by the practices of Somatic IFS, getting training and supervision in touch, and becoming informed by professional ethical guidelines provide important guardrails to protect against the use of inappropriate, unethical, or harmful touch.

With touch supported by the underlying practices, coming from Embodied Self, the part of the body that we touch knows we are literally "in touch" with it. This direct relationship can facilitate the part's willingness to share its story of physical neglect or abusive touch encoded in sensations and blocked or frozen movement impulses. The stories may not yet have words, but they still need to be heard. The touch from Self can be reparative to wounds of deficient attachment or violations of touch. We don't advocate the use of touch to reenact the trauma the client experienced without the client's Self energy present. Because of the sensitivity of the process and the possibility that the client's parts could see the therapist as the perpetrator, we track somatically for the response of the parts to the touch and for the presence of Embodied Self energy. Attuned touch may be the missing experience that parts have longed for, for decades.

Touching from the Embodied Self—with the permission of the client's parts, grounded in the other practices of Somatic IFS—can be from the Self of the client, the Self of the therapist, or from a safe individual or being in an imaginary scenario. Many IFS therapists are relieved to hear that the practice of Attuned Touch does not require them to do the touching. In fact, often when I ask clients whether their part wants touch from me, from them, or from both of us, they reply that the part is content with their touch alone. This signifies for me that the part feels safe with the client. Somatic IFS is in keeping with the IFS premise that the central agent of healing is the client's Self energy. When that is not available, the Self of the therapist steps in until the path is cleared for the Self of the client, and then the part is held in the exponential power of Self.

Imaginary Touch

Imagined touch between the part and the Self internally may be the only kind of touch many therapists utilize. It is safe to assume that every IFS therapist has used imaginary touch and has found it to be a natural and effective part of their therapy, especially with young, vulnerable parts. In Somatic IFS, often it is all the part needs. Imaginary touch may be used with parts not yet ready for direct physical contact.

Even imaginary touch releases oxytocin. Clients can imagine that they or someone safe is holding, hugging, or caressing young parts in their inner world, bringing many of the benefits of actual physical contact. They may see or sense infants reaching out to them from a crib or hospital bed. They lift them up and hold them securely in their arms. Young vulnerable parts may leap into their laps. Protectors, freed of their tasks, may hold hands with or lean into the Self for much-needed rest. Imagined physical contact plays a role in many internal scenes.

> Steve tunes in to the tension in his stomach and finds a ten-year-old boy who is desperate to be held but is afraid.
>
> **SM:** Let him know you understand he is afraid. Ask him if there is a way he can get some touch that won't be so scary.
> **Steve:** He is open to trying to touch hand-to-hand with me.
> **SM:** Good idea. Let me know what happens.
> **Steve:** He touched my hand. Now he is hugging me. My belly feels calmer. Now he needs to back off a little. He's about a foot away from me. This was new for him, different. He thinks it's too good to be true. For now he wants to sit outside in the sun. I tell him he can come back any time for a touch or a hug, whatever he needs.

When I work with a client by phone, imaginary Attuned Touch has an important place in a Somatic IFS session. Theresa is an IFS therapist who was consulting with me by phone. She shared her insecurities and dread about her work. Her parts were aching with the desire to help people in her care but were overwhelmed with the responsibility that was clearly beyond their capacity. She remembered how her father would comfort her frequent night terrors as a child, holding her tenderly. Little Theresa would cling to him and he would hold her just as tightly. He did not tell her she had nothing to fear. He didn't tell her to go back to sleep. He just held her, and she felt his understanding and compassion. Theresa entered those early memories and imagined being held by her father as they both held all her little insecure parts in between them. She said they were creating a cradle of love to hold all her parts. She told me tears were running down her face, and soon I could hear her sobbing.

The Client's Self Touch

Often the client's spontaneous touch literally points to a part. The therapist notices, and invites the client to notice, their hand automatically tapping their chest or their heart, stroking their forehead or cheek, or rubbing their finger against their thumb. Bringing physical contact to a part inhabiting the body can help maintain a focus on the part. When the client attends to the tissues under their hand, they can get a direct sense of the tension, the blocked energy, the inner chaos. Their touch can speak to the part, saying hello to unloved or isolated parts in the body: "I'm here with you now," "I'd like to get to know you," "I see how hard you are working," "I'm sorry," "What do you need?" "Can I help you let go of this?" "How is it now?" The client can put one hand on the place in their body they feel their Self energy and the other hand on the part that needs the compassion, or hold both parts of a polarized pair. For clients who have had their touch boundaries violated, self touch is an alternative—and a prerequisite—to receiving touch from a therapist.

Sometimes touch contacts a part when the other verbal and nonverbal approaches can't reach it. Bill was a successful, high-profile leader in business and also adept at many healing techniques. His industrious parts had served him well, but sometimes they got in his way. When he sent his breath to the fear in his stomach, it neither helped him connect his frightened part nor eased the stomach tension. With my suggestion, he used his hand to explore the tightness—the variations, the depth, the parameters. Then he said with surprise, "He doesn't feel so alone anymore!" His hand had conveyed the message "Yeah, I can tell how tightly you are holding on."

The therapist checks to make sure the touch is from the client's Embodied Self in order for the touch to be healing. For example, when one client brought mindfulness to her slapping of her thigh, she found a part telling her thigh she hated how fat it was. As the part separated, she explored the textures of her skin and underlying tissue and sent a message of apology to her thigh for her critical part. Another client seemed to be bringing Self energy through her touch to a part in her shoulder, but it was not having any effect. We realized the part touching was a thirteen-year-old caregiver part that lacked confidence, and once it stepped back, her Self-led touch helped her shoulder to soften.

For clients with sensory-processing issues, such as hyper- or hypo-touch sensitivities, therapists can help them experience tactile sensations by slowly and gently offering opportunities to feel different textures in the office environment. They can name and notice the textures and their responsiveness to them. Clients who have experienced touch violations need to know they are in charge of what they touch and how they touch. Self touch can bring awareness to places in the body that have become dissociated and open up blocked channels of energy. The parts residing there may have an aversion to pleasant touch, regarding good sensations to be dangerous, confusing, or potentially activating of exiled traumatic experiences. These parts may gradually begin to associate safety, comfort, and pleasure with what they feel through their fingers or hands.

The Therapist's Touch

Just as with the client's touch, the therapist needs to be in Embodied Self. Parts with an agenda to fix, correct, protect, or otherwise get our own needs met, parts with fears or insecurities, are recognized and asked to move into the background to be worked with later as trailheads to our therapist parts or our own touch histories. I typically use my own touch only after a stable, trusting, resonant relationship is established and I am assured that the client has some access to their Self energy. My touch might be in addition to the client's touch. My hand atop my client's is a physical representation of the therapeutic relationship in IFS—my Self energy joining with and supporting my client's Self energy so the part feels held, perhaps literally, by both of us. I will ask the client if there are any parts that have any concerns about me making physical contact. Especially if there have been touch violations in the client's history, it is crucial to touch only with permission from all the parts. I let the parts know that—under no circumstances—will the touch become sexual touch, and I check to learn how the parts respond to that statement. With touch neglect as with touch abuse, often there are polarized parts. Knowing I can't entirely rely on the words of permission, I track for somatic clues and my own intuition.

I have found that when I am literally "in touch" with the part, it is more willing to share its story, especially with early physical neglect and touch violations. The first inherent impulse is to reach out. When that is unsuccessful, as we have learned, the ANS overrides this first automatic response from the ventral vagus nerve and kicks in the more primitive responses. The stories encoded in sensations and frozen movement impulses can be contacted through touch. They may not yet have words, but they can be heard. Touch can restore that social-engagement impulse of the ventral vagal nerve in addition to other impulses that have been exiled.

This next session shows how my touch was used to find and focus on a part, listen to its story, unburden it, and restore its lost qualities.

Janet is being sexually harassed by a work colleague. She feels trapped and afraid of the consequences of stopping or reporting the harassment. As she speaks her hand repeatedly touches her chest. Bringing awareness to this place she is touching, she feels a strong burning sensation. She alternates between fear and anger and distraction, and she is not able to focus on any of these parts. Thinking my touch could help her stay focused, I ask Janet to check inside to see if her parts are OK with me placing my hand on the place that is burning—either on top of her hand or just my touch alone. She wants just my touch.

I leave my chair and sit close to her on the sofa. I again ask her to go inside to make sure that all her parts are OK with this touch. She says they are all fine. I let her know she will be in charge of the touch. I establish my vertical alignment, breathe into my heart, and slowly move my hand toward her chest. Her face and body relax slightly as she feels my touch. She directs me to make a few slight changes in my touch to best contact the burning sensation.

In the tissues under my hand, Janet notices a slight contraction. I tell her I feel the subtle movement as well. As Janet stays with this sensation she finds a part that is trying to get away. I say, "Let my touch tell the part I am listening. I understand it wants to get away." I feel the tissues begin to soften, and Janet feels it too. She is curious to get to know more about this part that is wanting to get away.

With Janet's Self energy more present, I slowly take my hand away from her heart, and Janet's hand replaces mine. "Tune in to this curiosity you are feeling and send it through your hand to this part in your chest. Let it know you want to hear what it has to tell you." With one hand on her heart, Janet speaks of wanting to get away from this man, while her other arm begins to make a weak pushing movement. Janet wants to be able to express this more fully in her body. I place my hands on her feet to help her feel more grounded. "Where do you feel this urge to push him away?" "Right here," she says, touching her stomach. I bring my hands to this place to support the movement impulse. She begins to push in space, and then I provide a firm presence to push against. Janet's whole body shows the satisfaction of being able to express her power.

Janet goes inside again to find the part that was afraid to confront this colleague. She is able to listen to its early experiences of powerlessness and unburden its fears. After this significant unburdening, she finds rest in my arms. She is glad to realize she can say no to unwanted touch while also accepting and appreciating wanted touch.

Attuned Touch and Boundaries

This session with Janet highlights the issue of touch and personal and professional boundaries, which is at the core of Attuned Touch. The perception of being violated or nourished by touch is dependent on the culture and personal history of the person being touched as well as the context. Our clients' histories almost always include some perception of their personal internal or external space being invaded, if not violated. When there has been physical or sexual abuse, there has been a violation, a rupture, a shattering of the integrity of a person's boundaries. Physical assault, combat, serious accidents, even medical procedures rupture the skin, the boundary between the inner and outer worlds. The experience of violation is registered in the somatosensory system and recorded in the limbic brain. Attuned Touch can repair these ruptures.

The protectors in the traumatized client's system play a crucial role. Protector parts have a variety of responses to the person's boundaries being violated. They may assume their chance for safety lies in establishing extremely rigid boundaries concerning touch and physical closeness. Their strict control of boundaries binds their body and mind in chambers of isolation. Other protectors are on high alert, hypersensitive to sensory experiences and avoidant of touch. Still other protectors might concede to touch but then numb the body or dissociate from the experience. A client locked in a dorsal vagal state of collapse will likely have a lack of boundaries, or diffuse boundaries, with an inability to gauge whether or not they want touch, to know what kind of touch, and to distinguish between abusive and safe touch. The client's system may alternate between these two poles of rigidity and laxness. Vulnerable parts may poke through the protective shield. The client might comply with the suggestion of touch, or even seek it out, and parts may try to reenact the trauma, casting the therapist in the role of the perpetrator in an attempt to tell their suppressed story.

The burdens associated with boundary violations affect the various modes of perception, and unburdening them is a delicate process. We bring consciousness to the unconscious perceptions. The ingrained neuroception of danger in mind and body is recognized and followed to the places in the body where parts whose boundaries were shattered reside. Much of the witnessing of the wounded parts' stories is in the implicit, nonverbal realm, involving breath, voice, and eye contact. We earn the trust of the dissociative or hypervigilant protectors. They come to be able to perceive the level of safety in the present regarding physical touch.

We might begin to restore healthy touch boundaries with imaginary touch, and then with the client finding a place that can tolerate physical touch. The client might start with their hands or arms, trying different places, pressures, strokes. The client may expand the touch to include other places in the body while staying in the present moment. As they touch, they are alert to parts that arise—both protectors and the vulnerable ones awakened by the touch. Touch can calm the hyperaroused exiles and restore ventral vagal involvement to the system. The client eventually discovers a level of safety in being in their body.

When the client indicates they are ready to experience the therapist's touch, the therapist checks to see if there are parts that may not yet be ready, and, if so, addresses their needs, concerns, and fears. With permission from the protectors, touch can be received and integrated in small doses—always with the client's Self present, directing the touch. Soft strokes to the arms or back speak directly to the insula and other limbic structures to calm them and communicate safety and emotional support. Knowing they are in charge of the touch, they tolerate, then accept, then come to appreciate being touched. Gradually, healthy touch boundaries are reinstated. Clients can use touch exercises outside of sessions to stabilize their nervous systems so they can continue to heal from their boundary violations.

Attuned Touch and Sexuality

Sexuality is enormously significant in our life, and the topics of skin and touch, necessary touch, touch abuses, and boundaries all intersect with this topic. In our highly sexualized and touch-deprived culture, physical contact, especially pleasurable or sensuous touch, is often confused with sexual innuendo. Confusions with sexual and nonsexual touch, and conflating all touch with sexuality, have contributed to both the abuses of touch and the prohibitions of touch in psychotherapy from its earliest days. When I first informed my father about my professional entry into the field of bodywork, he asked in horror if I would be working in a "massage parlor," fearing his daughter was announcing her intention to become a prostitute. He would have been a bit more reassured if he had confused the term with auto repair.

The practice of Attuned Touch can heal sexual wounds and restore the client's ability to find pleasure in sex.

My client Judy wants to improve her sexual relationship with her husband. She feels sad that she can tolerate only a very little skin-to-skin contact with him. When in close contact her parts feel trapped, afraid they will be manipulated into having sex against their will. Judy says the experience is "gut-wrenching." Her part fears her husband will leave her if she doesn't give in to his desire for weekly sex. This fear leads to a young part who believes she will die if she says no. Her part leaves the place where she is trapped and joins her in the present.

Judy holds her stomach as she tells her part she doesn't have to do anything she doesn't want to do. Her gut relaxes. Her part gets curious about why in the world she wants to have sex. Judy tells her sex can bring her love, happiness, sensuality, and more energy. That all sounds good to her part, but this part isn't sure she can get these things from sex. After some more physical holding from Judy, she experiences a bit of this love, happiness, and sensuality from the touch. Judy says the part let her know she is ready to try to feel this good stuff with John.

Judy is able to engage in sex with her husband and is finding some enjoyment as well as relief from his pressure. But she says this "love making" is not giving her a sense of loving or being loved. The part not feeling loved is a frozen four-year-old who was molested by the person she most counted on to love her and protect her, her father. This part is the same part that showed up in our earlier session. As she responds to Judy's compassionate presence and offer to help, she says she wants to be held. She first sits on Judy's lap, then she leans into Judy's chest with her arms around her. This part is clear about exactly the kind of touch she wants. She doesn't want to be stroked. She wants to lean and be held. She begins to thaw out but deep inside is still frozen; she is very guarded and doesn't want to be rushed. Judy tells her she is really glad she found her, that she has been looking a long time for her, and again tells her she doesn't have to do anything she doesn't want to do.

Judy: It feels like our bellies are connecting and there is some warmth there. Now she is starting to cry.

SM: Good, she is thawing out on the inside.

The part shows Judy an image of the molestation, and how bewildered she felt, and that this was when she froze.

SM: Thank her for showing you this image, and let her know you can take that image, like a photograph, and she can just stay with you, belly to belly.
Judy: She is tearing up the photo. Now she is burning it. She feels warmed by the heat of the fire.
SM: Let her feel the warmth, take it deep into her body.

Judy's belly feels looser and her part says hers does too. Her imaginary touch and Self touch has significantly healed her trust. The test and ultimate healing of the restoration of her trust in others, especially regarding erotic touch, will be outside of our sessions in her closest intimate relationship.

Conclusion

I am completing the writing of this book in the early days of the COVID-19 pandemic. We have been advised to shelter in place and practice social distancing, which of course means avoiding touching. It is uncertain what the long-term effect will be on our behaviors around touch. At this moment in time as we restrict even our hugs and handshakes, I have found comfort from these words in a poem written by Lynn Ungar on March 11, 2020, called "Pandemic": "Do not reach out your hands. Reach out your heart . . . Reach out the tendrils of compassion that move, visibly, where we cannot touch."[19] I look forward to a time when touch is no longer dangerous to our health and we can confidently benefit from the healing effects of loving, attuned touch.

The use of touch for healing is as ancient as the need for healing of both mind and body. Touch for healing has also held a polarized and often exiled role in our culture's history and has sparked a hundred-year-old controversy in the psychotherapeutic community. The practitioner in Embodied Self harnesses the healing potential of this intervention while avoiding harmful touch—not only sexual touch but subtler forms of unhealthy touch. The practices of awareness, breathing, and resonance provide a foundation for the toucher to be in a state of Embodied Self, and they link this practice of Attuned Touch with healing and spiritual practices throughout the ages.

Somatic IFS celebrates the reemergence of the practice of appropriate, ethical touch from its place of exile, where it has lain hidden in the shadows of fear and shame because of its association with sexuality, abuse, and violation. We understand that the violence in society and touch abuses in the therapy office are related to touch neglect and abuse, and that the path to prevention lies in repairing these wounds through touch. Rather than avoiding touch, we can use touch to awaken these dormant, usually wordless, and often imageless clues to our psychological and cultural burdens where they are available for repair.

Attuned Touch happens within the context of many multilayered associations with touch. We explore the complex layers of emotions, beliefs, and behaviors embedded in our inner systems as we unpack our touch histories. We consider the sexual, touch, and trauma history of the therapist and client, the culture and religion of the therapist and client, and the gendered or hierarchical nature of the therapist–client relationship. The Somatic IFS practices underlying Attuned Touch offer the tools for assessing appropriate safe boundaries around this powerful practice and for reading and responding to the messages from touch. Each of the four elements or all of them together support the practice of Attuned Touch, and they link the healing practice of Somatic IFS with healing and spiritual practices throughout the ages.

Although Attuned Touch may not be appropriate with all clients, in some instances touch may be the most direct and effective of all the nonverbal forms of expression. As a reciprocal sense, touch simultaneously gives and receives information through the somatosensory system. Even more than tone of voice, facial expression, or posture, touch tacitly conveys Embodied, Relational Self energy from client or therapist. Attuned Touch can repair the wounds from too little of the right kind of touch and too much of the wrong kind of touch, restoring our birthright of sensory aliveness.

Perhaps the flow of information through our sensorimotor system can affect a field beyond the individual's brain. Just as culture influences our experience of touch, and as touch wounds have negative cultural effects, perhaps person-to-person, reparative, nurturing, affective touch can positively influence the wider culture. In the area of healing, perhaps touch can be the bridge that joins the two artificially separated fields of body and mind.

Touch, like the connective tissue it contacts, is a tangible manifestation of the web of life. Each human being—from their earliest experiences bouncing off the uterine walls, being squashed in the birth canal, and emerging into the world to be held by their elders, to becoming an elder and welcoming new members into their arms—represents a segment of humanity that may span a time line of two hundred years. Touch is the warp and weft of the fabric of our life. Being attuned to what, who, how, and why we touch and are touched is essential to life.

The following Code of Ethics from the United States Association for Body Psychotherapy is a useful guide for the therapist concerning the ethical use of touch in psychotherapy. The exercises assist with imaginary touch, self touch, and using actual touch with a client during the steps of Somatic IFS. The survey on the use of touch as a psychotherapeutic intervention clarifies your experience with and considerations of various kinds of therapeutic touch with clients.

USABP CODE OF ETHICS*

VIII. ETHICS OF TOUCH

The use of touch has a legitimate and valuable role as a body-oriented mode of intervention when used skillfully and with clear boundaries, sensitive application and good clinical judgment. Because use of touch may make clients especially vulnerable, body-oriented therapists pay particular attention to the potential for dependent, infantile or erotic transference and seek healthy containment rather than therapeutically inappropriate accentuation of these states. Genital or other sexual touching by a therapist or client is always inappropriate, never appropriate.

1. Body psychotherapists evaluate the appropriateness of the use of touch for each client. They consider a number of factors such as the capacity of the client for genuine informed consent; the client's developmental capacity and diagnosis; the transferential potential of the client's personal history in relation to touch; the client's ability to usefully integrate touch experiences; and the interaction of the practitioner's particular style of touch work with the client's. They record their evaluations and consultation in the client's record.

2. Body psychotherapists obtain informed consent prior to using touch-related techniques in the therapeutic relationship. They make every attempt to ensure that consent for the use of touch is genuine and that the client adequately understands the nature and purposes of its use. As in all informed consent, written documentation of the consent is strongly recommended.

3. Body psychotherapists recognize that the client's conscious verbal and even written consent for touch, while apparently genuine, may not accurately reflect objections or problems with touch of which the client is currently unaware. Knowing this, body psychotherapists strive to be sensitive to the client's spoken and unspoken

---

* Source: https://usabp.org/USABP-Code-of-Ethics

cues regarding touch, taking into account the particular client's capacity for authentic and full consent.

4. Body psychotherapists continue to monitor for ongoing informed consent to ensure the continued appropriateness of touch-based interventions. They maintain periodic written records of ongoing consent and consultation regarding any questions they or a client may have.

5. Body psychotherapists recognize and respect the right of the client to refuse or terminate any touch on the part of the therapist at any point, and they inform the client of this right.

6. Body psychotherapists recognize that, as with all aspects of the therapy, touch is only used when it can reasonably be predicted and/or determined to benefit the client. Touch may never be utilized to gratify the personal needs of the therapist, nor because it is seen as required by the therapist's theoretical viewpoint in disregard of the client's needs or wishes.

7. The application of touch techniques requires a high degree of internal clarity and integration on the part of the therapist. Body psychotherapists prepare themselves for the use of therapeutic touch through thorough training and supervision in the use of touch, receiving therapy that includes touch, and appropriate supervision or consultation should any issues arise in the course of treatment.

8. Body psychotherapists do not engage in genital or other sexual touching nor do they knowingly use touch to sexually stimulate a client. Therapists are responsible to maintain clear sexual boundaries in terms of their own behavior and to set limits on the client's behavior towards them which prohibits any sexual touching. Information about the therapeutic value of clear sexual boundaries in the use of touch is conveyed to the client prior to and during the use of touch in a manner that is not shaming or derogatory.

SURVEY ON THE USE OF TOUCH AS A PSYCHOTHERAPEUTIC INTERVENTION

(If you wish, you can send your responses to this survey to me at susanmccon @gmail.com to add to the data I have already collected.)

Gender identity _____

Age _____

Professional identity _____

1. For what purposes do you use *your touch* therapeutically with your clients?

   ✓ To greet or say goodbye

   ✓ To access, contact, focus on parts

   ✓ To support the process of differentiating parts from Self

   ✓ To witness the parts' body stories

   ✓ To contain or comfort parts flooded with emotion

   ✓ To assist parts in a dissociative state to ground, reorient to the present

   ✓ To facilitate the process of unburdening

   ✓ To assist with the integration of restored qualities

2. In what ways does your client's gender, age, race, or clinical issue affect your use of touch?

3. Are there other considerations that affect your decision about touch?

4. Have you experienced clients misinterpreting your touch?

5. Do you know of clients who have experienced touch abuses in therapy?

6. Which of your parts have concerns about touching your clients?

7. Do you have any burdens from early touch abuse or neglect that might hinder Self-led touch with your clients?

8. Do you notice your clients spontaneously touching places in their own bodies?

9. Do you suggest your clients use their own touch to work with their parts?

10. Do you use imaginative touch with your clients?

EXERCISES

Imaginary Touch

PURPOSE To provide a part with a Self-led experience of receiving imaginary touch.

INSTRUCTIONS:

1. Remember a time or times when you received touch that was welcome, loving, connecting, and healing. Let the memory develop with sights, sounds, smells, and sensations. Notice your sensations as you stay with this memory. You can return to this memory at any time during this exercise.

2. Invite a part that would like to receive this kind of touch right now to emerge. If a part arises that has burdens from abusive or painful touch or a distressing neglect of touch, ask that part to wait until you have the support of a therapist.

3. As the part emerges and you sense it, see it, hear it, or feel it in your body, notice how you feel toward it. When you feel curious, friendly, and open, send that energy to the part and notice how the part responds.

4. Notice how close you are to the part. If your part is OK with more closeness, ask the part if it wants to come closer to you or if it wants you to come closer. Ask the part if it would like physical contact.

5. Let the part know it can have exactly the kind of physical contact it wants, that it is in charge of what kind and for how long. Give this touch to the part in your imagination, as you see or sense this part.

6. Notice what happens to the part as it receives the physical contact. If there is a verbal meaning associated with the touch, include the words with your touch. If the part would like to feel your physical touch, make contact with it where it is in your body.

REFLECTIONS:

1. Which part emerged? How did it respond to the touch?

2. Ask your part what could help it reinforce its experience of receiving loving, healing touch. Art, words, an object, your own touch?

3. If you have a history of unresolved touch abuse or neglect, consider making a plan to work with the parts in a safe environment.

Self Touch

PURPOSE To learn how an individual's touch can access a part that wants reparative touch and how the touch can provide the part with the Self-led touch it needs.

INSTRUCTIONS:

1. Awaken the awareness in your hands, such as by touching them, rubbing the palms of your hands together, moving them, becoming aware of the line between your heart and your hands.

2. Slowly brush your hands over your entire body. Attend to both the different sensations in your hands and the various sensory responses to your touch all over your body.

3. Notice places on your body where your hands linger or return to. Consider if there is a place on your body that might like more physical contact.

4. Bring your focus and your open curiosity to this place in your body to see what kind of touch it might want.

5. Breathe into your heart, and send the breath of love from your heart to your hand. Then make contact with this place in your body with the intention to simply be present. Let your hand meld with the surface of your skin.

6. Listen with your hand to responses in the skin, muscles, fascia, bones, blood, rhythms, energy. Notice any sensations in the

place in your body you are contacting. You might experiment with different kinds of touch, different pressures, different strokes, different paces.

7. Listen with your hand and your heart to any emotions, thoughts, or images in response to your touch.

8. This touch may have invited a part inhabiting your body, or it might be that this place in your body is needing the touch.

9. If it is a part, find out more about the part, invite it to show itself more fully in thoughts, emotions, words. Let your touch communicate your presence, your understanding, your willingness to get to know this part. Engage in verbal or nonverbal communication to discover what kind of touch can bring connection, comfort, or healing to the part.

10. Stay fluid with your touch as the part changes or moves around in your body. When your part feels complete with the touch, stay connected with it energetically as you gently disconnect physically.

REFLECTIONS:

1. Make a note or a drawing to indicate the place on your body that wanted touch.

2. What kind of touch did this place prefer?

3. Were your hand and heart able to "listen" to this place?

4. Was it a part that showed up in your body wanting the touch? If so, what did you learn about this part? Did you get a sense of its experience with touch?

5. What kinds of touch did your part want?

6. What happened when the part received touch from you in Embodied Self energy?

7. Did any parts arise that were concerned about your touch?

Working with a Client: Attuned Touch and the Six Fs

PURPOSE   To illustrate how Attuned Touch can facilitate each of the steps of the IFS model when working with a person in the client role who is exploring their touch history or who wants to work with a part receiving touch from another person.

INSTRUCTIONS:

The steps are not strictly sequential but are a guide to the person in the therapist role working with a client's parts concerning touch. It is important that the client has some degree of Self energy available during the session while receiving touch from the therapist; if not, the therapist works with the parts until they can trust what is happening in the present moment. The therapist may set boundaries on the touch for reasons of safety, ethics, or their own touch histories.

1. **F**ind the part. The client may share a touch memory or a part that wants to experience receiving touch from another person. It may be a part that didn't receive enough touch or the kind of touch it needed, a part that received the wrong kind of touch, or a part that was not able to be in charge of the touch and wants to repair the hurt. Ask if the part is showing up in the body. The therapist finds any of their parts that have concerns about the touching and asks them to step to the side and jump back in if they feel uncomfortable.

2. **F**ocus on the part. If the memory is triggering to the client's inner system, many other parts may jump in. If the part (and other parts) is OK with contact, either therapist or client touching the place in the body where the part resides can help keep the client's attention focused on the part. The focusing touch communicates a willing, open presence. If the client's parts can't step back, this indicates the protectors need to be worked with first. The therapist works with these parts with the six Fs, with or without touch.

3. **F**lesh out the part. Therapist and client invite the part to show itself in its fullness—possibly emotions, words, images, thoughts. If the part is not yet evident somatically, the client's touch may be able to locate it.

4. How do you **F**eel toward the part? The answer to this question from the client allows the therapist to assess if there is some degree of Self energy available in the client. If not, it is another opportunity to work with parts protecting the vulnerable ones that were hurt by touch prior to working directly with the core injury. The therapist also checks inside for any parts that may obstruct the flow of Self energy through their hand.

5. Be**F**riend the part. Ask the client to check inside to see if their parts are willing to receive the touch—if no parts object, the therapist's touch can transmit the qualities of Self energy through their hand. The movement is slow, tracking the client's response, and the touch from the hand is similar to the movement of *yield*. The therapist communicates a constant presence through their touch. If at any point in the session the client's system becomes flooded by emotion, touch may help the client return to the present moment and provide a soothing, grounded presence— for example, touching the client's feet, arm, or hand or placing their hand on the client's back near the heart. The therapist is open to stopping the physical contact whenever the part or another of the client's parts requests it.

6. **F**ind out what the part wants you to know. The part may share its history, its job, and its feelings both verbally and nonverbally. The therapist's hand is receptive—open to any somatic information from the part's response to the touch. The therapist's touch responds to any perceived shifts by making slight changes in the amount of pressure and the kind of touch, getting verbal feedback from the client. If the part is sharing a painful touch experience, the therapist and/or the client may use touch with the six Fs to witness the part's story and to provide a reparative touch experience.

7

Embodied Self:
The Internal System Embodied

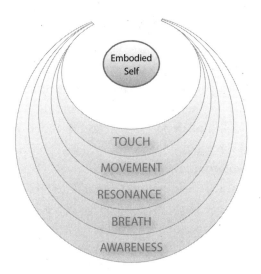

"EMBODIMENT" CAN BE DEFINED as the subjective experience of being in our body, being present to our moment-by-moment sensations and movement impulses. More fundamentally embodiment could be described as *being* bodies, as *being* our sensations and movements. It is the natural state of most animal species. These sensory abilities are adaptive. Interoception (the capacity to feel our body) and exteroception (the capacity to sense and make sense of the external world) have helped our species survive. Embodiment has allowed us to sense danger and to defend ourselves from it. Beyond survival, embodiment is a state where we are most alive, capable of feeling our joy, compassion, pleasure, and connection with others and the world around us.

It is clear that the internal family does not just exist in the brain—that both parts and Self are embodied. Mere days after conception, a handful of cells demonstrate creativity, communication, and collaboration. These few cells organize for survival, attending to the organism's needs for protection and nourishment. In the newborn, Self energy is palpable, as are its parts, as its distinct personality emerges. The infant's parts enter the world with gifts of spontaneity, courage, intelligence, creativity, and sensitivity. Other parts lay dormant, manifesting when developmentally appropriate throughout the life span. The infant's Self energy, although deeply sensed, is largely latent, concealed in a vulnerable and defenseless body. The young body and brain are not yet equipped to actualize the inherent power of Self energy. For the most part, the quiescent qualities of Self energy lie dormant, awaiting maturity of the nervous system and the rest of the physical body to manifest Self's fullest potential to lead the internal system.

Meanwhile, if the external environment doesn't provide the necessary loving care and protection, the parts may become so battered and shaped in all sorts of ways that their original, shimmering, pristine gifts get distorted or buried. By the time the individual has developed the physical and emotional resources to speak up, to attempt to defend themselves against life's wounds, their parts don't believe Self energy exists. They don't believe the outside world welcomes and supports them. They can't hold onto a belief in their worthiness. Yet the parts still echo with the sacredness of their origin. The echo can be heard in the parts' positive intentions.

In the body we find it all. The burdens are in the body, the original gifts are in the body, and the qualities of Self energy are in the body. The most holy qualities of our parts and Self buried deep in our body are a source of wisdom, strength, and healing. With Self energy in its embodied state through the practices of Somatic IFS, our buried resources are discovered, excavated, and reinstated. Our parts are freed from the roles forced upon them and can resume or assume harmonious, collaborative roles and relationships with each other and with Self. Their functions, their tasks, and their characters emerge in ways and times appropriate to the current situation. Our inheritance is restored.

Embodiment, as well as Self energy, is on a continuum. Those of us who have had unburdenings through IFS therapy or other healing modalities, and who have a body, brain, and nervous systems functioning well enough to support and express the qualities of Self energy, are among the more fortunate to live our life more or less at one end of the continuum. But Embodied Self is a dynamic state. We move along the scale of this continuum moment by moment and day by day. Speaking personally, in stressful situations my parts take over and Self energy seems no more than an elusive concept. My degree of embodiment shifts as well, moment by moment. I may ignore messages from my body needing to move or rest or get attention, as if my body were an annoying pest. The marvelous mutable play of sound, light, shadow, movement, and texture surrounding me is shut off from my senses. Over time, the pull toward the disembodied, parts-led end of the continuum has weakened. I waste less time there, and I more easily and quickly move back toward the Embodied Self end.

Yet none of us has attained our fullest potential. I have glimpses of the possibilities of full embodiment as I watch my dogs, who, even though domesticated, quiver with delight when they sense the waves of Lake Michigan crashing on the shores, and when they catch the scent of numerous wild mammals as they romp in the woods. They are so enthralled by the world's delights that, freed of their leashes, they dash joyfully in infinity-shaped loops. Not encumbered by the more complex cortical processes of the human brain that analyze and distract, or hang on to fears, resentments, and outmoded beliefs, my dogs nearly overwhelm me with their exuberant glee each time I return after having abandoned them. I also have glimpses of the reaches of Embodied Self energy from books or documentaries about the remaining nomadic and indigenous people whose survival depends on it. Every unburdening leads us closer to the fullest potential of Embodied Self.

The Unburdened Embodied Internal System

IFS trainer Mariel Pastor has contributed to our understanding of the characteristics of our parts when they are unburdened: "Parts work more harmoniously together . . . The inherent gifts of each part are more available, weaving in and out consciously."[1] Many of Pastor's portrayals of unburdened parts are embodied qualities, evoking images of young people dancing, laughing, happily working and playing with each other. The descriptions that follow are from "The Unburdened Internal System" mandala she created with Dick Schwartz:

- Unburdened Protectors: Many parts may be released from their protector roles, while others will effectively protect only when needed.

- Unburdened Firefighters: Signal Self directly when stress levels are high. Have effective self-soothing activities and diversions. Add spice to life with passion and adventure, healthy risk taking and humor. Advocate for fairness and stand up to injustices. Lend courage and confidence to act bravely in challenging situations.

- Unburdened Managers: Offer a balanced approach to daily responsibilities. Effective and competent, able to collaborate and encourage other parts and people. Advocate for growth and contributing talents. Can be lovingly parental and nurturing to other parts and people.

- Unburdened Exiles: Tender, sensitive parts with childlike curiosity and delight, advocating for connection and care. Secure with Self as primary caretaker, feeling freer to reach out to others. Offer intuition about others' feelings. Enjoy being open and trusting.

Pastor's depictions of these unburdened parts include some of the words portraying Self energy that begin with the letter C—curious, creative, connected, centered, calm, compassionate, courageous, confident, and clear. This indicates that when freed of the effects of its wounding, no longer divorced from Self energy and so acting in extreme ways fueled by fear and isolation, the part has restored its relationship with the Self of the individual. This energy so permeates its being that the Self of the part is awakened. Unburdened parts do not become rehabilitated, obedient parts of the personality that have learned to behave and follow the Self's lead. Their functions and character within the system are infused with their own Self energy.

The IFS model recognizes the parallels between the internal family system and both smaller and larger systems. Just as the internal family system has parts and Self, parts have parts and Self as well, and those parts have parts and Self, and so on, although in clinical practice it usually is sufficient to work at the level of parts having parts and Self. The systemic aspect of IFS is applicable to larger systems. Whether the IFS therapy is focusing on the individual's internal family, the couple, the family, or larger groups, it takes into account the reciprocal influence of both smaller and larger systems. I refer the reader to the excellent chapter in Schwartz's second edition of *Internal Family Systems Therapy*, "Applying the Model to Social and Cultural Systems," which looks at our cultural legacies such as racism, patriarchy, materialism, and homo- and transphobia and offers a vision of a Self-led country:

> Our eyes and ears would open to exiles and the destruction we are inflicting on the planet. This awakening would expedite our efforts to reverse climate change, economic inequity, and discrimination. We would offer treatment rather than punishment for destructive firefighters . . . We would value relationships over material possessions and power.[2]

Schwartz ends this chapter with the inspiring view that healing intrapersonal systems can heal larger systems:

> And since human system levels are interconnected, Self-leadership at any level helps to heal all levels. We believe that each client who unburdens helps reduce the burden load of the planet, allowing all of us to have a little more access to the Self.[3]

Somatic IFS addresses more specifically that the individual burdens concerning the body often have their roots in racist, patriarchal, and heterosexist attitudes transmitted through societal institutions. These attitudes cause damage to bodies, including loss of life. The cultural and intergenerational burdens embedded in the institutions of a racist society result in injury to Black bodies, including violence and death. The traumatic legacy of over four hundred years of racial injustice based on the body's appearance, to be seen not as people but as property, is embedded in the institutions and practices in our society as well as in the body-mind of individuals. Patriarchal institutions perpetuate violence against women, as women, too, have been considered the property of men. The most extreme bodily result of this cultural legacy is physical abuse, sexual abuse, and loss of life. Although having attained equality on many levels, women are burdened by being viewed as objects, and by objectifying their own bodies as a means to success in our society. For people identifying as queer, living in a society that pathologizes those whose gender identity and/or sexual expression lies outside of the socially constructed binaries is an obstacle to embodiment. The LGBT community experiences violence and death because of a homophobic and transphobic society. More generally, trauma from physical and sexual abuse, from neglect, from childhood or adult chronic illness and physical disabilities, and even from accidents and surgeries can often be traced to cultural norms and institutions.

Whether we are a member of the dominant culture or of the oppressed groups, the burdens embedded in our culture's institutions gradually and insidiously serve to extinguish our access to Embodied Self energy. Young children's freedom to cry loudly, to squirm, giggle, and skip, is crushed. White heterosexual males absorb the cultural mandate to limit the expression of their vulnerable emotions for fear of being humiliated, beaten up, or rejected. We may feel shame toward our bodily secretions, excretions, and smells, and revulsion toward bodies that are disabled, ill, or old, whether they are others' or our own. Our physical ailments are either ignored, taken to a professional, or are finally a reason to get the attention we crave.

There is evidence that the cultural burdens connected with racism, sexism, and heterosexism are shifting. The internal work we do as we heal from these societal wounds leads to Embodied Self energy. The inherent resiliency is also evident in both black and female individuals and subcultures. The #MeToo and Black Lives Matter movements have arisen in response to societal objectification and devaluing of female and Black bodies.

As we embody Self energy, we can more effectively work to heal the wounds of our society. We are more impervious to the statements and actions of the culture. The practices of Somatic IFS restore our subjective view of our body from the inside out. This consideration of similar patterns within patterns is consistent with the view of many mathematicians and scientists that the entire universe—from the subatomic, atomic, molecular, cellular, organismic, to the interpersonal and cosmic levels—displays fractal properties. Fractals are objects or systems in which the same patterns repeat at different scales and sizes. Many natural phenomena are fractal to some degree. A head of romanesco broccoli and a snowflake are examples of fractals. This theory considers that our universe may be an enormous, seemingly infinite, fractal structure where the whole is expressed even in the tiniest parts of the pattern and vice versa.

Somatic IFS considers the fractal properties of the internal family on both the conceptual and the physical levels. The human body displays fractal properties, with parallels within systems and within structures of the body. One example is the branching of the pulmonary system—from bronchi to bronchioles to alveoli—where the whole is encoded in each part and all parts together compose one interconnected whole. We find fractal design in the organs—kidneys, liver, pancreas, and brain. The function and structure of the cell membrane is repeated in the skin and in the fascia that envelops the organs, muscles, blood vessels, and nerves. The cell's cytoskeleton, which connects every part of the cell from the membrane to the nucleus and all the organelles, echoes the musculoskeletal system and connective tissue of the body. This cytoskeleton and the continuous web of connective tissue, along with nervous, cardiovascular, and other tissues, together contribute to the body's form. They also conduct the flow of energy and information within each cell, within the body, and outward to the environment and from the environment to the innermost parts of the cells. These structures work synergistically, forming a living matrix, a continuous interconnected semiconductor network.

The fractal nature of our universe is one of the defining characteristics of a hologram, where every part of a hologram contains all the information possessed by the whole. The human body can also be viewed as a hologram existing in a much larger hologram we call our universe. The idea of a human as a microcosm of the universe and each part of the body as a microcosm of the whole human body is embedded in much of Chinese and East Asian philosophy and is the framework for traditional Chinese medicine. For example, there are acupuncture points on the feet and the ears that are connected to various other parts of the body. A foot reflexology chart somewhat resembles an image of the human body. Artists, philosophers, and healers over hundreds of years have recognized the fractal and holographic properties of the human body. Unlike Western science, which attempts to understand physical phenomenon by dissecting, compartmentalizing, and studying its separate parts, a hologram teaches us that dissection simply leads to smaller versions of the whole, and that everything is also fundamentally interconnected and part of the larger whole. This view pertains not only to space but also to time.

A recent experiment conducted in Geneva testing quantum theory separated two subatomic particles by a distance of seven miles and found they responded simultaneously to a stimulus applied to just one of them.[4] The behavior of these particles is explained by physicist David Bohm, who was a protégé of Albert Einstein and one of the world's most respected quantum physicists. These two particles actually aren't separate, he says. Their separateness is an illusion. Perhaps this view suggests that our perception of particles as individual entities is incorrect, and that our perception of ourselves as individual entities is also not in line with reality but filtered through our senses. Einstein himself is famously quoted as saying "Reality is merely an illusion, albeit a very persistent one."

Every part of a hologram contains all the information possessed by the whole because it isn't actually a separate part. This is the simplicity that lies at the core of all the complexity and diversity we perceive around us. This view that contradicts our commonplace experience, that all things are infinitely interrelated and influencing each other—essentially that we're all one—has enormous implications.

The implication for Somatic IFS is that our inner system is an indivisible bodymind system infinitely connected with every other level of system in the universe. We identify different aspects of the internal system just as each of us claims a unique individual identity, while remembering they are useful constructs as we navigate our perceived "reality." We are a physical body but we are also a consciousness residing in a holographic field of energy and information that then directs, guides, and continuously rebuilds the physical form. The Embodied Self is woven into every level of our inner beings and in our relational web, and it is evident in the Field of Self energy. There is available to us a continual flow of energy and information from all these seemingly separate levels. The "whole in every part" nature of a hologram provides us with the idea that each part of the bodymind internal system is inextricable from the much larger consciousness of Field of Self. The only thing seemingly separating our parts from this Field of Self is their burdens. The "most persistent" of these burdens is the illusory belief that we are separate.

It is clear from all this that the result of psychological healing does not mean the separate aspects of the internal family dissolve into an indistinguishable mush. There is an integration within the system, but it is not because the parts disappear or merge into a bland sameness. Rather, without the burdens restricting and distorting their perceptions and behavior, parts are free to recover their original gifts, to fulfill their purpose, and to engage in constructive, collaborative relationships. A healed internal family is a microcosm of individuals in a healthy, loving family (or, if that is hard to imagine, a group whose members love and respect each other and are dedicated to a common cause) who exhibit similar qualities while they uniquely contribute and collaborate for the good of the whole. Each part's leadership is respected even while the core Self of the individual—influencing and influenced by the parts, and connected with the wider Field—guides and leads and unifies.

We are primarily holographic fields of energy and information and secondarily physical beings. Unburdening releases blocks in the bodymind system, allowing the body to repair and heal itself. The body can maintain a high degree of coherence, supporting the extraordinarily complex bodily processes.

The body's informational field has within it the blueprint for health, theoretically able to heal any disease. We just need to eliminate the blocks.

The late Rockefeller University physicist Heinz Pagels, like many other theorists, believed that quantum physics is a kind of code that interconnects everything in the universe, including the physical basis of life itself. He had the understanding that he (and therefore presumably *everything*) embodied the principle of life that transcended death. In his book *The Cosmic Code: Quantum Physics as the Language of Nature*, Pagels, an avid mountain climber, wrote of a dream he had of falling, terrorized as he fell into the abyss:

> Suddenly I realized that my fall was relative; there was no bottom and no end. A feeling of pleasure overcame me. I realized that what I embody, the principle of life, cannot be destroyed. It is written into the cosmic code, the order of the universe. As I continued to fall in the dark void, embraced by the vault of the heavens, I sang to the beauty of the stars and made my peace with the darkness.[5]

Pagels was killed in a climbing accident six years later.

The thirteenth-century mystic poetry of Mevlana Jelaluddin Rumi conveys many of the principles of quantum physics that Pagels wrote about. One poem fragment tells us that it is in our body that we can find the peace we seek:

> There is a life-force within your soul, seek that life.
>
> There is a gem in the mountain of your body, seek that mine.
>
> O traveler, if you are in search of That,
>
> Don't look outside, look inside yourself and seek That.[6]

Many of his poems speak to each of the Somatic IFS practices of awareness, breathing, resonance, movement, and touch that help us mine the gem, the life force in the mountain of our body. I include a poem fragment at the end of the following discussion of each of the practices as another voice to convey an aspect of the fully embodied, Self-led internal system that is the goal of Somatic IFS.

Having explored each of the practices as a path to Embodied Self, we will now consider how, unfettered by burdened parts, the state of full embodiment that is our birthright is expressed in each of these practices. Our cells reverberate with awareness, our breath is full and easy, our movements are fluid, and our entire body facilitates resonant connections.

Embodied Self Is Expressed in the Five Practices

Somatic Awareness

When in a state of Embodied Self, we are exquisitely aware of our body. Our body pulses with awareness. Our senses are receiving the flow of information from the outside world. Our every cell effervesces in aliveness as it communicates and coordinates with other cells and with its surrounding fluid to accomplish its unique mission. Each organ is pulsing in its own rhythm, creating together with the other body systems a persisting symphony. With an awakened awareness of our body, we embody many of the C words that describe Self energy.

One of the primary aspects of Self energy is feeling **centered.** When in touch with our center we know where we are, who we are, and who we are not. Many of us point to the center of our body to show where we feel Self energy. Some say it is a cylindrical core; others indicate one particular point—their heart, their navel, their stomach. The physical experience of being centered involves our proprioceptor cells as well as the structures in each cell that have an awareness of the action of gravity and our relationship to our vertical alignment. Unburdening may have literally changed our center of gravity. Centered physically and conceptually we have a sense of equanimity and balance. We are unattached to outcomes. When we temporarily get knocked off center, we feel it viscerally, and through our body we find our way back to our center. We tune in to the actual physical center of our body to access our Self energy and become the quiet "I" in the center of the storm. When we stay centered in our body, the storm loses its velocity and is restored to a state of calm.

Another of the C words accessed through Somatic Awareness is **connection.** Connection is evident on every somatic level in an unobstructed bodymind system. Our fascia, which is literally encasing our body as well as touching every other system through its abundant sensory nerves, is an example of this embodied connection. Each of our trillions of cells is busy exchanging information and communicating with other cells, with the larger systems of the body, and so on, to infinity. This quality of connection is evident in the embryo and it persists throughout our life in our cells and in all our body systems. Each system of the body is autonomous yet interdependent, connected with every other system.

With Somatic Awareness we sense the connections among the members of the embodied internal family. Body and mind are connected, all parts of the body are connected with each other, and parts are connected with each other and with Self. Aware of our body, we more easily connect with our parts and how they use our body sensations to perform their roles and to communicate with us. We are aware of the subtle messages from parts in our internal system sent through our body sensations. They feel our connection. They don't need to get extreme in hopes of being noticed. Grounded in our bodily experience unfolding moment by moment, the inherent wisdom embedded in our body is available to us.

Connected internally, we also connect externally. Through our body we reach out to others and concretize the relational web. We are grounded and supported by others every step of the way. So many have walked the earth before us and we walk in their footsteps. We feel our connection with the universe and all of life, with our ancestors and with future generations. With gratitude to Earth for its gifts, we pledge to live in harmony with it and to preserve its health for future generations.

Through our sensorial bodies we are aware of our relationship with the earth and other life forms on the planet. We know where we stand. We walk in **confidence.** The core of the earth speaks to us of belonging, security, and stability. Our confidence grows from our appreciation of the earth's abundant support, from how seeds we have planted have flowered and been harvested during our lifetimes. Like the earth, we know the rhythms and cycles of change, the mountainous heights and the deep darkness of caves. Somatic Awareness and the earth element have become a firm dependable anchor in the face of tumultuous emotional energies. Our confidence is contagious. Our confidence encourages our clients to find safety and support from the earth, to trust that even their deepest secrets and darkest fears can become fertile soil for tender new seeds to flourish.

This dynamic ability we inherited from ancient ancestors to sense danger as well as to open to pleasure is available to guide our actions. We reach deep into the earth and our roots spread wide. The dust of our ancestors, our teachers, and our mentors nourish us. In our life we express our gratitude to the earth and its people for all the gifts.

Rumi tells us, "There are a thousand ways to kneel and kiss the earth." We can then push off from our knees to reach into the space beyond, segueing to the next practice: "You are in your body like a plant is solid in the ground, yet you are wind."

Conscious Breathing

This second practice of Somatic IFS also portrays the **connection** quality of Embodied Self energy. With the element of air marrying the element of earth, we are living out our awareness of our place in the world. Anchored to the earth through our seat and our feet, we open to the space above and realize our vertical alignment, our connection to above and below. We are not only connected, but we are *the connector* between the earth below us and the infinite space around us. Our body can act as a lightning rod to ground chaotic energies from without. The earth gives us solidity, while the air reveals that at the most basic level we are mostly empty space. Breathing unites the solid matter of our body with energy, the seeming void that appears to be nothing and yet might be everything, that might be as crucial to our spiritual lives as the invisible oxygen is to our physical lives. Breath connects the unconscious and the conscious, guiding us from our preoccupation with the past or the future back to the present moment.

The act of breathing connects us to our interdependence with all living things, with our mutual dependency on the life-sustaining gas of the thin layer surrounding our Earth. We breathe in this precious air and breathe out the illusion of our separateness. This synergistic exchange of gases is the dance of our essential unity and interdependence. Our breath connects us human beings to the animate world of both plants and animals. In Embodied Self, we strive to protect the air from pollutants and the trees from logging and burning. Through the act of breathing, each cell is connected with the outer environment in a continual exchange of oxygen and carbon dioxide, connecting inner and outer worlds, uniting us, if not with the entire world of aerobic life, at least with the inner systems of our clients. Lying between the introspective practice of Somatic Awareness and the relational practice of Radical Resonance, Conscious Breathing links the intrapersonal, interpersonal, and transpersonal systems.

In our breathing we find our inherent **curiosity.** When in Self we easily tap into our curiosity as effortlessly as we breathe. We breathe in the spaciousness from the Field of Self energy, and we transmit that spaciousness as we breathe out. We breathe curiosity in to whatever arises in our consciousness, and we breathe out the sound "hmmm . . . ?" We continue to breathe in our curiosity: "Where in my body is this emotion/belief?" "How am I feeling toward it?" In the "hmmm" of the long, slow exhale, we experience a letting go, an opening to the unknown. Whether we imagine making the sound or actually hum, the vibration of this humming sound resonates in our head and in our chest, dissolving any confusion or efforting. After the "hmmm," something new may emerge out of the void. We may find spaciousness, or information, or simply the enjoyment of breathing, of humming, of not having to know. As therapists, in the spaciousness we remember our client has Self energy. When truly present from a place of wonderment, our curiosity takes us to a sense of awe, as "hmmm" changes to "aaaahhh." The curiosity that arises on our inbreath ignites our imagination, our intuition, and our inspiration to support us in our healing relationships.

When we breathe in curiosity rather than rehashing our conditioned perceptions, on the outbreath we access another of the qualities of Self energy,

clarity. When I took my Buddhist precepts I received a new name, Chong Gak. My Zen master told me both words were different ways of saying "clear." If I can indeed claim any attainment of clarity, I attribute it to bringing consciousness to my breathing. There was not much else to focus on while continually asking my parts to step aside while sitting in stillness and silence for days at a time. Meditation teachers tell us that as our body becomes still, the sediment of our stirred-up, murky mind eventually settles out, leaving our mind and body clear. With a part reluctant to step aside, I met it on the inbreath with a gentle query, "What is this?" and on the outbreath with an expansive "Don't know." Eventually clarity arose.

Jack Kornfield, one of my favorite authors and teachers who bridges the spiritual and psychological realms, draws on the insights of leaders of Western and Eastern spiritual communities in his book *After the Ecstasy, the Laundry: How the Heart Grows Wise on the Spiritual Path* that are relevant for "After the Unburdening."[7] When the parts affecting the breathing are unburdened, we find becoming conscious of our breath helps us navigate the complex real-world challenges in our work, our health, our aging, and our relationships. When parts arise out of habit to meet these challenges, awareness of how these parts affect our breath brings a restoration of the calm and clarity, leading to a creative response to the challenge. Breathing brings clarity on a physiological level as well as maintaining emotional clarity.

The respiratory system cleanses the body of its cellular burdens. When our bodymind system is like the air on a clear day, our senses are sharp, our thinking is expansive and precise, and we know what we feel and express it lucidly. Conscious Breathing supports our clarity of speech. The most direct expression of our bodily knowing might be silence. We know when to speak and what to say when there is a clear channel to our bodily wisdom. We discover that clarity is a magnet. Kornfield shares a famous quote by William Butler Yeats, who speaks of the transformative power of this practice: "We can make our minds so like still water that beings gather around us that they may see their own images, and so live for a moment with a clearer, perhaps even with a fiercer life because of our quiet."[8]

Conscious of our breathing we find a state of **calm.** Bringing consciousness to this largely unconscious practice influences the involuntary nervous system, affecting our heart rate, blood pressure, digestion, and metabolism. Whether we simply become conscious of this largely unconscious activity or engage in a specific breathing technique, our full, easy breathing gently rocks us in the rhythms of in and out, giving and receiving, filling and emptying, echoing the rhythms of nature. When in the grip of parts our energies tighten and narrow, become denser, more constricted. The rhythms of respiratory and cellular breathing create calm and spaciousness within our body and mind. Each inbreath brings new possibilities, new life. Each outbreath allows us to let go of what we no longer need, making space for the new.

Compassion is also available to us through our breath. The oxygen from our breath goes first to our heart, nestled in between our lungs. Our heart powerfully pumps oxygen-rich blood to our cells, and it transmits equally precious compassion throughout our body, and we breathe out compassion. We breathe in Self energy from the surrounding space and breathe it out into the relational field. Our breath supports our Embodied Speech to convey this presence through our tone, our pitch, our rhythms. We don't claim this presence is *ours* but is simply *presence* flowing through us like the air to those in the world in need of healing. The precious air enlivening our heart ushers in the relational realm of the next practice, Radical Resonance.

Rumi tells us the "breath of love" can take us "all the way to infinity."

Radical Resonance

It takes **courage** to go "all the way to infinity." Courage derives from the Latin root *cor,* meaning heart. From our heart flows the courage to dive into the deep waters of relationship. When fear and desperate need no longer encumber our relationships, our heart no longer needs to be walled off by layers of protection. Our senses don't need to be dulled. We find possibilities of deeper intimacy. We are free to resonate with our external world, including other living beings. Experiencing the physical and emotional vibratory energy emanating from every seemingly solid material substance, we begin to comprehend the reality of the relational web we are a part of. Beyond concepts of self and other, mind and body, matter and energy, there is simply the invisible evidence that we are all equally imbued with spirit.

As our heart leads us to deeper intimacy, our body-based attachment experiences are revealed. Parts that have habitually navigated the complex, often tumultuous world of relationship may be at a loss. Many of the wounds we suffered were experienced in this horizontal realm of relationship, and they have worked diligently to keep us from further harm and to let their hurts be known. In particular they may have experienced the energetic frequencies of those around them to have been overwhelming and chaotic. They may have learned very early to shield their openness. Although recognizing that their beliefs and behaviors are outmoded, these parts may feel disoriented, pink-slipped, and aimless. These parts are not yet in sync with the new vibrations.

We bring the courage of our openheartedness to them. Courage is not the absence of fear but walking with the fear. We are willing to resonate with these parts, to allow them to merge their energies with our own. We are impacted emotionally and vibrationally while simultaneously staying connected to the vibration of Self energy. As we do this, just as one in-tune instrument can bring an instrument playing slightly off-key into tune, resonating with the frequency of a part can bring that part into coherence with the frequency of Self energy. This coherence is reflected in neural, chemical, and energetic patterns in the body. We also tell our parts that there may still be situations where their screens, shields, and shutters will be necessary. Restoring our resonant capacity does not mean we have forfeited our ability to modulate our receptivity. Sensing when it is safe and desirable to be open is an aspect of Radical Resonance.

A famous Zen story depicts an ultimate courageous stance in the face of fear and the transformative power of courage. As the story goes, when word got out that a murderous thug was coming to town, all the people of the village except for one headed for the hills. When the killer heard that this one person had the audacity to stay, he pounded on their door. When the person opened the door, the man pulled out his sword and yelled, "Do you know who I am? I am someone who could cut you in two without blinking an eye!" The person looked into the eyes of the man and calmly replied, "And do you know who I am? I am someone who could be cut in two without blinking an eye." At that, the murderer sheathed his sword and turned away.

In our heart also lies our capacity for a true, deep **compassion.** Our heart feels warm, open, and tingly, and the energy beams outwardly. The roots of the word compassion mean "to suffer with." Kwan Yin is known in Buddhism as the Goddess of Compassion, and her name means "She who hears the cries of the world." It is said she not only observes the suffering but *suffers with* in order to heal. She is an example of simultaneously living inside the skin of a tormented being while also being differentiated, holding the pain in an infinitely large container.

Although the etiology of compassion implies suffering with the person in pain, compassion is not a painful experience, but rather a rewarding one, as shown in some recent research shared by Dick Schwartz in *Internal Family Systems Therapy*. A large-scale study by Tania Singer and her colleagues with the Max Planck Institute in Leipzig, Germany, focused on how the effects of mind-training practices such as meditation might influence not only individual well-being but also social issues of peace and justice. One of their functional MRI findings showed that empathy and compassion share different brain networks. Empathy activates pain circuitry, while compassion activates the reward circuitry. Compassion is a presence, while empathy is an emotional merging. Our heart swells with compassion as we resonate with another's pain. It has the effect of uplifting us rather than dragging us down. We discover that our whole body, as well as the space around us, provides a large enough container to hold seemingly intolerable pain.

Our heart-felt, radically resonant receptivity is transmitted wordlessly and received vibrationally by the client's bodymind system. Parts' burdened beliefs dissolve. Relational ruptures are repaired. Habitual behaviors lose the reinforcement from the old synaptic firing patterns. The vibrations of myriad dissonant parts come into coherence as the brain and body are rewired. The unburdening, coupled with the energetic transmission of Self energy, frees the client's Embodied Self to become the secure attachment figure for the client's young parts. The Embodied Self of both therapist and client creates an exponentially amplified frequency of compassion. The parts come to know the biological and psychological reality that they are a part of a larger whole.

The Self-led quality of **calm** is also a hallmark of a resonant relationship. We sense this quality in our body—our breath, our heart rate, our relaxed musculature. This calm state in our brain has a vibrational frequency that can be measured. This rhythm, perhaps not coincidentally, happens to be the same amplitude as the rhythm of Earth. The planet's rhythm, a set of electromagnetic wavelengths that has been reliably measured since the 1960s, which has come to be called "the heartbeat of the Earth," is known as Schumann's resonance. This state of calm is remarkably different from the apparent "calm" that results from suppressing and controlling our reactivity, or when collapsed on the sofa or immobilized in our chair. It is not a static state but as dynamic as the deep ocean waters whose surface may get ruffled by the wind. In the state of Embodied Self energy, in a resonant relational state we appear calm, sound calm, and transmit calm to others' nervous systems even as we talk, move, and interact.

We may glimpse the reality beyond our sensory experience of our inseparability. Although we continue to function as separate individuals, and to relate to others and to our internal system as having separate, discrete components, just like the Geneva experiment demonstrated that the subatomic particles were not separate, we too can live out that reality. Our concepts of therapist and client, self and other, can be held lightly in a larger awareness. We can expand beyond notions of interpersonal, intrapersonal, and transpersonal healing too as we live out a harmonious relationship with other human beings, with all living beings, with the planet, even with the universe. Our resonant bodies become channels of the energy and information flowing along all the seemingly discrete, hierarchical levels of our universe from the subatomic to the galactic. The healing potential of resonant relationships is enormous.

Rumi's poetry speaks of this non-dual, resonant relational field: "when the soul lies down in that grass, . . . language, ideas, even the phrase 'each other' doesn't make any sense."

Mindful Movement

The power of our **creativity** evidenced in our moving bodies is truly deserving of our awe. The body's creativity, plasticity, and potency is evident from conception onward as cells multiply and differentiate to form constantly evolving structures, communicating and collaborating to meet new needs and challenges throughout our life. We yield in the watery world of the uterus. We attach to the wall and float and swim. We play with various movements. In Embodied Self we access the creative, playful potential of movement that is our birthright. Throughout our life, the body in motion is the source and the means of expression of our creativity. Movement, associated with the element of fire, ignites our creativity and gives it expression. We don't need to stay stuck or collapsed in the face of anything life delivers to us. Dilemmas and conflicts are recognized as an opportunity for creativity rather than paralysis. We don't need to memorize techniques as therapists. Innovative, appropriate interventions arise within the relational field. We might even rise from our chair and invite our clients also to stand, to lie down, to crawl, to allow the stories to find expression in movement. We resonate and mirror their movements.

We have looked at how revisiting embryological development can uncover the natural movements that express our true nature before later disruptions occur. Traveling along the space-time continuum to our earliest incarnation, we reconnect with our inherent creativity and power to protect and nourish ourselves. We connect with the movement of pulsation, which is at the core of life. We have focused on the movements of yield, push, reach, grasp, and pull for indications of interference with the inherent unfolding through movement, either acquired from developmental trauma or inherited or epigenetically transmitted. With traumatic wounding we have brought mindfulness to the first attempts to escape to safety, to the adaptive reflexes to fight or flee, followed by the collapse if the body's resources are overwhelmed. Gradually, mindfully, slowly, and safely revisiting these movements buried in our neuromuscular systems has allowed the movement story to unfold. This leads to an unburdening of the movement patterns as well as the perceptions, beliefs, and emotions. In this way Mindful Movement becomes an agent of transformation of the client's limbic brain and body systems, stabilizing the physical expression of the internal shifts with awareness and mindful repetitions. The restored flow of the life force is expressed in new movement patterns of grace, strength, and flexibility.

When in Embodied Self, our movements express our **confidence.** Our restored confidence is reflected in our open, expansive posture, in our gait and gestures, and in every move we make. We can stumble, lose our footing, lose our balance, and we quickly regain it. Like courage, our confidence does not rest on hoping things will turn out OK or eliminating everything that is not OK. The source of our confidence is a knowing that everything is already all right. We have within us all we need. Our body is a storehouse of confidence that we can draw from when we face the unknown. We can feel confident in our own skin, just as we are, regardless of our size, age, or abilities. We don't have to know what lies ahead. We confidently walk in the dark, sensing only what is under our feet. We no longer have to make ourselves small enough or invisible enough, nor puff ourselves up.

Rainer Maria Rilke, in a poem in *A Book of Hours,* writes that God is telling us to keep moving, no matter what. In his poem God tells us to go to the limits of our longing in order to embody God, to "flare up like a flame and make big shadows I can move in."[9] We don't turn away from our longing, fearing disappointment or failure. We go to its limits. Where do we go to find it? Is it, as Rumi suggested, a "gem in the mountain of our body"? When we find this gem in our body, God tells us to "flare up like a flame." The movement, the behavior, the activities fueled by our Self-led longing take us to surprising places in the world where our light casts shadows large enough for God's movements. As we move into the world with confidence of Embodied Self, Rilke continues to voice advice from God: "Let everything happen to you: beauty and terror. Just keep going." We just keep moving throughout our life with sure and confident action, living out our purpose, one step at a time.

Rilke's poem echoes Rumi's: "Dance, when you're broken open. Dance, if you've torn the bandage off. Dance in the middle of the fighting. Dance in your blood. Dance when you're perfectly free."

Attuned Touch

The aspect of **connection** associated with Self energy is most fundamentally and concretely expressed through the practice of Attuned Touch. Those of us who remember when we had to pay for long-distance calling may recall the old AT&T commercial encouraging us to "Reach out and touch someone," depicting tearful scenarios of separated people with a backdrop of emotion-laden music now connected through long-distance phone connection. Although phone and other devices do their part to keep us connected with others, direct physical contact is far more impactful. The connection through touch travels through the sensory nerves of the skin all the way to every part of the brain, bringing the message "I am with you as you are with me." Connected with our body, supported by the wider Self Field, and in a resonant connection with the person being touched, parts are held in the exponential power of Self. We somatically track the responses—before and during the touching episode—for nonverbal responses to the touch within our own body and the body of the person being touched. Our touch changes almost simultaneously with the response.

Throughout our life we all long to touch and to be touched, and our physical and emotional well-being depends on it. My urge to become a clay artist came from a desire deep in my belly to "touch others" with my art. Moving and breathing I wedged and molded the clay; the imagination and creativity lying dormant in my body found expression through the clay. I loved the various sensations of working with my hands as clay met water, as wet clay was dried by air, and as dry clay was transformed by fire. Messages from my body shaped the clay under my hands, and the finished pieces brought something from within to the outer world. These pieces touched others, sometimes enough for them to want to buy them. At some point, though, I returned to wanting to touch others, and I decided to do it more directly, which I did as a bodyworker. Sometimes, more than anything, we need to give and receive actual touch.

This direct communication through the somatosensory system of both individuals may be the most potent and effective of all the forms of implicit communication between parts and Self, being literally in touch with the part. Touch, our first language, tacitly conveys Embodied, Relational Self energy from client or therapist directly through the skin, the outer layer of the brain. The energy flows through the vast network of fascia and nerves, a tangible manifestation of the web of life coursing through each of our individual bodies.

The act of touch from Embodied Self has no agenda, just **curiosity.** When we make physical contact, Attuned Touch—unlike some forms of bodywork or medical palpation—has no expectation of finding something wrong, of changing or correcting whatever we contact. The attitude conveyed is simply one of presence. Simply being present we are open to receiving the subtle implicit language of the body communicated through the flesh. Touching a place in the body, with the permission of the client's parts, where a part is residing communicates a message of open curiosity: What is it that is wanting to be heard that perhaps my hands can hear? What is it you are wanting to feel from me that you may be able to take in only through my touch? Our natural curiosity emanates from our hands and our voice. The one being touched may be able to trust the message from our hands more than from our voice. Our hands know how to be an open, compassionate channel for parts. Whatever we perceive through touch—tension, flaccidity, emptiness, fragility, melting, softening, opening—our hands continue to communicate a willingness to be present with it as it unfolds.

Attuned Touch conveys the **calm** of Embodied Self as touch travels from skin to brain and to every cell. As the story of physical neglect or abusive touch encoded in sensations and blocked or frozen movement impulses unfolds, it awakens what has lain dormant in the tissues. The tactile sensation of safe, connected, respectful touch travels along the afferent nerve pathways to restore the ventral vagal state of social engagement to the system. This calm limbic state travels along the efferent pathway to soothe

the hyperaroused exiles embedded in the tissues. The emotionally dysregulated parts can unblend as the effects of touch slow heart rate, reduce blood pressure, and unleash a stream of healing chemical responses, including cortisol and neuropeptides. Attuned Touch, whether it is imagined, from the client's Self, or from the therapist, conveys the somatic message to the parts that they are safe and supported. Safely held, they are calmed emotionally, physically, socially, neurologically, and perhaps spiritually. When the experience of touch has been associated with pain or abuse, Attuned Touch can establish a new message, that of being calmly, safely connected.

Just as culture influences our experience of touch, conceivably the healing power of person-to-person, reparative, nurturing, affective touch can reach beyond the individual. Research has demonstrated the correlation between touch deprivation and abuse and societal violence; healing individual touch wounds can hopefully have a positive impact on society. We are social creatures, and tactile experiences remain central to our well-being throughout our life. To the degree that the virtual community provided by social media has become a substitute for flesh-and-blood interactions, and that touch abuses in power dynamics receive society's tacit acceptance, the need for Attuned Touch transcends the individual. Attuned Touch has the power to heal touch wounds both intrapersonally and societally.

Somatic IFS celebrates the reemergence of the practice of appropriate, ethical touch from its place of exile where it has hidden in the shadows of fear and shame. Touch can awaken the dormant clues to our psychological and cultural burdens, rendering them available for repair, restoring our birthright of sensory aliveness as a people. Our individual and societal touch wounds, when not avoided or denied, can be the impetus for healing. When we "reach out and touch someone" from Embodied Self we reach into the very soul.

From Rumi: "I am not this hair, I am not this skin, I am the soul that lives within."

Case Examples Illustrating Use of the Five Practices

The three sessions that follow briefly demonstrate Somatic IFS with different clinical issues, making explicit how the five practices were integrated into the IFS model.

The Somatic IFS Practices Uncover Sexual Abuse

Diane was being troubled by some involuntary twitching in her pelvic floor. She thought the twitching might be related to some neuropathy from her chemo treatment. She goes inside to focus on sensations in her pelvic floor and instead notices a restless sensation in her legs (Somatic Awareness). While she stays with that, her legs begin to move in a jerky fashion (Mindful Movement). Rather than focus on the involuntary movements, I join her in breathing into our pelvic floors to help release the tension (Conscious Breathing and Radical Resonance).

As she breathes, Diane begins to rock. I join her in the movements (Mindful Movement). She enjoys the voluntary aspect of the movement, being in control of the movement rather than being at its control. Staying with the rocking, she uncovers a memory of being fondled by her doctor when she had a tonsillectomy at the age of four. Her shock and confusion at the time caused her to put a lock and key on those sensations in her pelvic floor. She realizes the twitching was this little girl beginning to break through the lock and key, trying to get her attention.

We both stand and Diane is aware of her feet, legs, thighs, and pelvis as she moves around the room (Mindful Movement). Her legs feel tingly and alive. They have more energy (Somatic Awareness). She enjoys the sensations in her pelvic floor as she moves her pelvis freely. I move with her and we both share what we notice in our bodies (Radical Resonance). Diane feels a line of energy streaming from her pelvic floor up toward her heart. She traces this line with her hand and laughs with delight (Attuned Touch).

The Somatic IFS Practices
Resolve Accident Trauma

As a young woman Elena had been in a serious accident that left her with chronic, debilitating headaches. It felt to her like a hammer was perpetually pounding the right side of her head (Somatic Awareness). Although she somewhat manages the pain with medication and tries to continue with her life as well as she can, she feels frozen in her body. She is curious to see if Somatic IFS can help restore what the accident had stripped from her—the joy and delight in moving her body. I notice her right shoulder and neck are held tightly and there is a stiffness and tentativeness in all her movements (Mindful Movement). There is an urgency to Elena's desire to rid herself of the pain, and I feel my body tense with effort. I let it go and focus on my heart. My compassion flows toward her as I think of what she has lost (Radical Resonance).

We revisit her memory of the accident, taking each moment of the experience slowly enough that Elena can bring mindful awareness to each body sensation that arises as she remembers the details of the accident. With each detail she recalls, we pause to notice the sensations in her body (Somatic Awareness). Gradually Elena's body begins to thaw. A slight movement begins in her spine, then increasingly includes her shoulders, neck, and arms. These first subtle movements progress into trembling, then to shaking. Tears begin to flow down her face. The shaking eventually subsides. She yawns and breathes more deeply. She moves her head and neck, looking around the room with a smile on her face (Mindful Movement).

I notice her legs are left out of all this wonderful movement and releasing. I invite her to tune in to her lower body to see if it wants to move as well. Elena tentatively attempts a very slight extension and flexion of her legs, but the movement is stopped (Mindful Movement). Bringing awareness to the stopping of the movement, she discovers a young, terrified part who is a short distance from the right side of her body. This young girl tells her about her father's hatred of weakness. The part fears that the weakness from the accident would arouse his hatred.

Elena reaches her arms toward the young one and draws her into her heart (Attuned Touch). She lets her know it is safe to move, that no one will call her weak. Elena's legs begin to tremble and shake. When they relax, she stretches her legs and then stands up (Mindful Movement). Her entire body is relaxed. She tells me the pressure in her head has lessened (Somatic Awareness). I see that her neck and shoulder on the right side are moving more freely (Mindful Movement). Having borne witness to the entire movement story of the accident restored the flow of energy in her body that will allow the natural healing process that had been impeded by her part's fear of her father.

With Elena, bringing mindful attention to the pounding in her head would not have brought release. Focusing on the pain would have unleashed a panoply of parts related to the sensation. Instead, bringing mindful awareness to each sensation that arose with each moment of her memory of the accident allowed the blocked trauma to release through the movements of trembling, shaking, yawning, and breathing. Awareness of the blocked movement in her lower body revealed her part that had been blocking her body's natural healing response. Imaginary touch to the part released the block, and the natural trauma response of shaking was allowed to flow.

The Somatic IFS Practices Encourage a Movement Story of Multiple Traumas

Sophie arrives at our session having had a recent encounter with a man whose behavior she found threatening. As she recounts the event, her breath quickens, her body becomes more tense, and her complexion pales (Somatic Awareness). I ask if she would be willing to temporarily leave the story to pay attention to the parts showing up in her body. She notices that her arms and legs don't feel connected to her core (Somatic Awareness). At my suggestion she stands up and takes a few steps into the room. She swings her arms and twists her core side to side (Mindful Movement). She says this movement helps her arms and legs feel more connected. As she is doing this, I find myself wanting to yawn and to move as well (Radical Resonance).

Sophie sits down and keeps her focus with her body. She notices a pull in the area of her solar plexus. Staying with the pull, she collapses down into the couch. Then she bolts upright as if to resist the collapse (Mindful Movement). We talk about these opposing movements perhaps indicating two polarized parts acting in her body. She lets the collapse take over more and more until she curls up in a ball (Mindful Movement). Staying in this curled-up position, she finds a part that blames herself for her childhood sexual abuse. It just wants to never get up again. She holds her stomach and imagines holding the little girl (Attuned Touch). Eventually the impulse to be upright emerges more naturally and she unfolds her body. Sophie then, at my suggestion, oscillates between less extreme versions of these two movements, guided by the rhythm of her breathing (Mindful Movement and Conscious Breathing). On the inbreath her front body extends. On the outbreath her front body flexes. I join her in the movements. We do this for several rounds of inhale and exhale. In flexion she tells her little girl it isn't her fault and that she is sorry no one saved her from the abuse. As her front body extends, she senses a part that is trying to help her survive both the sexual abuse and the physical abuse of her father. She feels the rigidity and compression of her spine (Somatic Awareness). She tells this part she is OK now and it can relax.

Sophie finishes telling the story of her encounter with the threatening man in a much more relaxed way. It is clear to her parts that Sophie is in Embodied Self. Sophie's part that jolted her upright, that kept her spine rigid, needs more attention. She exaggerates the tension of the upright posture (Mindful Movement). Although she no longer feels the pull into a collapse, she senses a lack of support in her spine and neck (Somatic Awareness). She leans against the couch, then asks me if I would be willing to sit back to back with her so she could feel my body supporting her (Attuned Touch).

As we do this, I synchronize my breath with hers. I can feel her breathing become fuller and slower and her back softening (Attuned Touch, Somatic Awareness, Conscious Breathing, Radical Resonance). When Sophie slowly pulls away and faces me again, her eyes are relaxed and there is a smile on her face (Somatic Awareness) as she tells me that was exactly what she was needing. She says she is glad this man threatened her because it gave her the opportunity to find parts related to her past trauma that were operating in her body but were hard to get to.

The Embodied Internal System as a Path to Oneness

IFS can be seen as a transpersonal or psychospiritual model. IFS has been shaped by many of the great intellectual, philosophical, and religious systems that all emerged around the same period of time, between the fifth and third centuries BCE. The teachings that arose from diverse Eurasian societies—from Socrates, Buddha, Confucius, Lao Tse, and the Hebrew prophets—shaped our culture to be more self-reflective. Jesus said, "The Kingdom of God is within you." Buddha told us, "Look within, thou art the Buddha." In the Upanishads is written, "Self is everywhere, shining forth from all beings, vaster than the vast, subtler than the most subtle, unreachable, yet nearer than breath, than heartbeat." Twenty-five hundred years later, their wisdom still informs and guides us and is a touchstone for our healing practices, including IFS. As Schwartz notes, "When our parts separate from the seat of consciousness (the Self) we discover what spiritual traditions have known and taught for thousands of years; that we have the resources we need to support and protect this vulnerable inner population with its awesome potential."[10]

Although it might seem obvious that looking within includes the body, its energies, and its sensory capacities, and that therefore a spiritual experience is an embodied one, much of philosophical thought and religious doctrine over the last centuries has considered the body to be an obstacle to the highest spiritual attainments.[11] The body has been seen as a hindrance to spiritual flourishing—a source of bondage, sinfulness, and defilement, tainted by karma. Sexual and sensual pleasure is demonized. The reward for a virtuous life will be to cast off this repulsive source of suffering and to finally rest in the bliss of a disembodied afterlife. This view has led to repression, asceticism, and the concept of exiling or sublimating the body to the "higher" goals of a spiritualized consciousness.

Rather than being an obstacle to spiritual attainment, the body is a path. Just as the concept of Self energy for IFS ushers in the spiritual dimension, even more so does Somatic IFS. Integrating mind and body sets the stage for the finale of the trinity of the integration of mind, body, and spirit. When mind and body are no longer separated in a false dichotomy, we

283

can experience this larger reality that spiritual masters speak of. Transcending dualism has a synergistic effect. Like when baking soda and vinegar are united, they dissolve and form a new substance that is released into the air—literally CO_2 and H_2O—the systems of body and mind unite to become bodymind and Spirit is released in effervescent energies.

Transcending the dualistic separation of mind and body as well as the trialistic separation of mind, body, and spirit, Somatic IFS brings all these human dimensions into a fuller alignment. Regarding the body as subject rather than object, and the Self as an embodied state, transports us to an embodied spirituality that views the body and its energies as essential for enduring psychospiritual transformation. Incarnating in material form, rather than being an obstacle to reuniting with the world of Spirit, is the route home to Spirit.

Becoming embodied is a life journey that begins in an embodied state, loses some of it, and hopefully restores it in time to gracefully allow our body to age, to fail, to fall apart, and to decay. Our body is the most mutable and protean of all the aspects of our beingness. Our body as it changes throughout our infancy, childhood, adolescence, adulthood, middle and old age is a testimony to the changing nature of the universe. Embodiment is not the end point of our existence. It is the beginning of awakening to spiritual wisdom.

We look within and, once our burdened parts step aside, we find the divinity within ourselves. It turns out this divinity that we call Self in IFS is a powerful, healing presence. Each Somatic IFS practice serves to restore and support our inheritance of being fully embodied and fully our authentic, essential Selves. We look without. We breathe in bits of each other with every breath we take. We touch our hands and our molecules intermingle. We realize we are much more alike in body and mind than we are different. We are all made up of earth, air, fire, and water and we all depend on these elements. We sense the web of connection that includes ourselves and every being.

When we try to talk about Spirit, or Self energy, it is as ineffable as bubbles that pop the moment we touch them. In trainings participants frequently want to talk about Self—what it is and what it is not. I find the longer we talk about Self the less we are in it. Very quickly into this discussion I move the group into an experiential exercise. It must be experienced to be grasped.

We tune in to notice different parts of our bodies, from top to bottom, front to back, from surface to depths. We notice our skin, our muscles, our fluids, our bones, our organs. We notice the rhythms of our aliveness. We notice our breathing, our movements. Our observing and witnessing deepens until we transcend having bodies to becoming our bodies. With this, we enter the realm of Spirit. As we more fully deepen into the experience of Embodied Self, paradoxically, we lose some of the sense of having a solid body with firm boundaries between the inside and the outside. Self energy, synonymous with Spirit or Soul, is ineffable. It may lose its anthropomorphic state.

In the following session, the client experiences his Self energy first as swirling energy and then he becomes one with the natural world of sea, sand, and sun. This client spent many years as a Buddhist monk and experiences parts and Self in somewhat different ways from most of my clients living in the West. This client has asked to be known as Windfarer and resides in an Asian country. He had learned about IFS and was so enamored of the model that he began a course of study to become a therapist so he could use IFS to help others heal. He wanted to experience the IFS model firsthand and was drawn to work with me for my somatic perspective and my Buddhist background. We began to work together online. He records and transcribes our sessions, so my report is verbatim in some places and in others is a summary of our conversation.

Windfarer felt his Self to be a swirling energy. As he stayed with this sensation, a part of him arose that had been triggered in his class when he felt he had not performed well. This part was looking for love, acceptance, and security. It had found this with his mother by being a "kitty cat," and with his peers by being the "King." This part striving for an excellent performance had paradoxically interfered with his performance when leading a group in class. The part said, "I need to cling onto something. I need to solidify. I need to get people on my side. I see an image of my mom judging, and I feel I have to be like a kitty cat, then I would feel secure."

As this part arose, Windfarer felt in his body a sense of solidity, a condensing and containment of his energies that told him he was losing his connection with Self energy. He did some ocean breathing to return to more Self energy. He was able to bring Self energy to this part. First his Self appeared as the swirling energy, and later as the sun, the sand, the sound of the ocean waves.

In this session, Windfarer did not see or sense his Self energy as his actual body but rather as energy, sound, and nature. He likened his experience of Self energy to what in Buddhism is referred to as "No Self," or the kind of emptiness described as enlightenment moments. Even so, he could talk with the part. I asked Windfarer to invite the part to show the attachment it has to doing well. The part showed him holding on, grasping, grabbing onto it. It shared that it was afraid of losing acceptance if it were to let go.

Windfarer: [*speaking to his part*] I see your true intentions. I wholeheartedly accept who you are. You always have a place in my heart. I am bowing toward you. I thank you for showing me of others in the world who are like you. You allow my heart to feel more compassion; to see more fully the range of where my compassion can extend. You have so much meaning to my heart and I bow to you.

As Windfarer looked at the boy's face, the face flashed into that of an old man, then a grown man, and then back to a young boy.

Windfarer: [*to me*] This part has a thousand faces. I bow to him. I feel my *prana* sinking deeper and deeper into my body. He is taking in my peaceful energy. Sweat is pouring out of my hands and feet. I'd like to get to know him better.
Windfarer's Part: I can be anyone. I can be anywhere. For everyone is me and I am everyone. Thank you for the sea, sun, and sands for showing me how I am part of all things and all things are a part of me.
Windfarer: So, are you no longer feeling lost and bewildered? No longer desire love from Mom?
Part: If I discover my true nature as being a part of everyone, then who is it that is lonely?
Windfarer: So you are really feeling that it no longer burdens you, does it? If you were not to have a mom who gives you warmth, you wouldn't feel lonely, or if you were in class without friends recognizing you to be a great therapist who achieved all these great deeds—even if you don't have that then you are still freed and secure?
Part: At this moment I am.

Windfarer: Can you feel me being here with you? Can you sense Us being with you?

Windfarer questioned his part because he wanted to make sure that this part had become unburdened simply by his presence, without the steps of witnessing, retrieval, and unburdening. He conjured up the original situation that had triggered his part—performing in front of his class—and this part continued to feel held in acceptance and compassion. Windfarer told me he felt like he was in a "wow" moment.

After a long, profound silence, Windfarer shifted into a conversation with me about his experience with Self energy and how it differed from his understanding of how most Westerners describe their experience. He wondered if there was a cultural bias that saw the Self as solid. His experience of Self is that the swirling energy was "bigger than stability." For Windfarer, Self energy is nothing and everything simultaneously.

Windfarer then shared with me an experience he had ten years ago of the realization of Oneness that put him on the spiritual path of Buddhism and, later, an exploration of transpersonal psychology. He told me that although his background in meditation and all the Buddhist teachings "kind of flashed in," during the session they didn't become an intellectual bypass. Although he could see how IFS works, he wondered if we hold too tightly onto the notion of parts instead of the larger reality that there is no body, no mind, no parts, no Self. He continued by considering that the root burden is the notion that we are separate from each other, an idea I too have been strongly contemplating. He explained his experience of Somatic IFS to me:

Windfarer: When I get to Self, I have so much respect for the part, and that transforms the part at that moment. My sense of acceptance is not only feeling good and accepting toward that part as being separate, but I am totally accepting that part at the level where I see that part is not different from me, and I am that part, and you are me and I am you. With that sort of acceptance, it gets at the root burden that we are separate. We differentiate the part from Self. We separate from the part. We differentiate, but then the differentiation dissolves. There is just judging, there is acceptance, it is all just, yeah, like there is clouds and the sun, the sand, the trees, the desert, me and Mom . . . If you get at the root burdens, they become all things and everything.

No Body, No Mind, No Self, No Parts?

With this client, as with many others, I have seen that freeing the internal bodymind system is a path to spiritual realizations. In Embodied Self they glimpse that beyond our ideas and concepts we are all equally imbued with spirit. Embodied Self, as a unity of mind, body, and spirit, is a transcendent state. We go beyond the limitations and constrictions imposed by our burdened parts. When truly embodied, Self energy paradoxically transcends our individual bodies. It goes beyond the limits of our skin, beyond the filters of our perceptive and sensory capacities.

Embodied Self is a hologram of the cosmic Field of Self. This coherent intelligence lying beneath or beyond the apparent material world exists in each one of us as well as outside of us. It supports and informs every level of the system and every level of the system contributes to it. Grounded in the earth, connected to the infinite energies from above, communicating with the Field of Self energy around us, we breathe it in, we breathe back into it. We move through this field, and it moves through us.

Supported and informed by this field, we look within and find our parts, each a hologram of the universe. We differentiate from the part in order to help it, while realizing it really is not separate from us or from anything. We differentiate from others, while holding a sense of our interconnectedness. We recognize in them their Embodied Selves as well as their parts, much like our own.

It seems that when we bring mind and body together, it not only opens us to the spiritual realm, but actually it causes us to begin to understand that all members of a system, from the subatomic to the interpersonal to the cosmic, are interdependent, interrelated, and indivisible. Conceivably the differentiations and definitions, the categorizations and the characterizations, are all in service to the attainment of this larger comprehension of the nature of reality. Just as we each claim an individual identity and as we identify different members of our internal system, perhaps we can regard these separate identities as useful and necessary constructs as we live out our life with the larger awareness that we are operating under an illusion of our separateness. Perhaps this "root burden" referred to by Windfarer, and researched, studied, and written about by Pagels, Bohm, Einstein, and many others, can be held in the conception of the larger Field of Self.

The practices of Somatic IFS lead us to the realization that we are a physical body but we are also a consciousness residing in a holographic field of energy and information. The qualities of Embodied Self are threads woven into the relational web and every level of our bodymind system. Energy and information flow in endless waves, continuously within all the seemingly separate levels of existence. We may glimpse the reality of our inseparability beyond our sensory experience. Although we continue to function as separate individuals and to relate to others and to our internal system as having separate, discrete components, just like how the Geneva experiment demonstrated that the subatomic particles were not separate, we too can live out that reality. Our concepts of therapist and client, self and other, can be held lightly in a larger awareness. We can expand beyond notions of interpersonal, intrapersonal, and transpersonal healing as we live out a harmonious relationship with other human beings, with all living beings, with the planet, even with the universe.

Embodied Self energy often eludes definition. In my experience as a trainer, the more we attempt to define what exactly Self energy is, the less we seem to understand it or experience it. Although Self energy cannot be located definitively in the body, when it is experienced and anchored in the body it becomes a known and lived experience. Many qualities that describe the state of Self energy, named for those of us who appreciate mnemonic techniques, begin with the letter C. These qualities—clarity, curiosity, courage, compassion, confidence, creativity, calmness, connectedness—are inherent, embodied states. The exercise that follows offers an alternative to describing with words this elusive state that is the goal of Somatic IFS—experiencing the qualities in the body. We have also found that, once experienced, this state is transitory. Although it is always there, parts obscure it—often when our systems and those around us most need it, unfortunately. The last exercise offers specific actions related to each of the five practices to help us and our clients quickly restore the state of Embodied Self energy.

EXERCISES

Embodying the Cs of Self Energy

PURPOSE   To experience the qualities of Self energy in the body. To find and release blocks to Embodied Self energy.

INSTRUCTIONS:

This exercise can be done individually (up to step 7) or in a group setting.

1. In any position, choose one of the named qualities of Self energy to explore it in your body. Where is it in your body? How does it show up? Particular sensations? What happens to the sensations as you stay with them?

2. What happens if you bring your breath into this place in your body where the quality shows up?

3. What happens if you allow this quality to move? What parts of your body want to move? Can you move through space with it?

4. What happens if you bring touch to this place in your body?

5. Can this quality be felt or expressed even more? What does it need to do that?

6. Are there any limits, any blocks to expressing or expanding this quality? Maybe the limits first show up as a feeling or a thought. Does your body participate in limiting this quality? What does this limiting part need to relax, to be OK with this quality being present and being expressed?

7. Staying in the position you are in right now, say aloud the quality of Self energy that you have explored, listening to others who may have explored the same quality.

8. Form a small group. Each member nonverbally expresses the C word they explored while others guess the quality of Self energy. Then verbally share your experiences.

9. Share in the large group.

REFLECTIONS:

1. Which quality did you select and why?

2. How were each of the five practices helpful in accessing the particular quality of Self energy you explored?

3. Which ones might help you quickly separate from a part and move more fully into Embodied Self energy?

Quickly Establishing Embodied Self Energy

PURPOSE To practice utilizing the practices of Somatic IFS to quickly re-establish Embodied Self energy.

INSTRUCTIONS:

Practice all the following exercises related to each practice. See how quickly you can do them and still get benefit. Do them right before a session. Consider inviting your client to do them along with you. Perhaps you will find one or more of the practices that most reliably and quickly anchors you in Embodied Self energy.

1. Somatic Awareness: Quickly scan your body, beginning with the places touching the floor or your seat and continuing up to your head and face, checking in with your skin, muscles, bones, and organs. If there are places in your body that hurt or feel uncomfortable, ask them to take a back seat for now, promising them you will return to them later. Let the weight of your bones help you settle into connecting with the earth.

2. Conscious Breathing: Take a couple breaths, noting the pace, rhythm, and any restrictions throughout your torso. Breathe into the restrictions and breathe out a long, full exhale. Breathe the spaciousness from around you into places in your body that feel constricted. Take one more breath into your heart. Feel the line of vertical energy making all the resources from the infinite Field of Self energy below and above available to you.

3. Radical Resonance: Expand your awareness to the person across from you. Notice any sensations that indicate obstacles to your open heart. Bring your awareness, breath, or touch to these blocks, bringing appreciation and reassurance to the parts protecting your heart.

4. Mindful Movement: Move slightly from side to side, front to back, flexion and extension, to facilitate your connection with above and below, your full, easy breathing, and your opening heart. Scan your body for any unnecessary muscular tension, especially areas where you know your parts hold tension. See if there is a slight movement you can make to release the tension.

5. Attuned Touch: Your hands can touch a place in your body where you have identified a part through these practices, communicating acknowledgment and reassurance to that part.

REFLECTIONS:

1. Did these exercises increase your Embodied Self energy? How do you notice it?

2. How long did it take you to do all of the above exercises?

3. If you have limited time, for example, before a session or within a session, which of the above practices would you use to help you quickly re-establish Embodied Self energy?

Notes

Introduction

1 Ken Dychtwald, *Bodymind* (New York: Tarcher Putnam, 1986).

2 Thomas Hanna, *Somatics: Reawakening the Mind's Control of Movement, Flexibility, and Health* (Cambridge, MA: Da Capo, 1988).

3 Richard C. Schwartz and Martha Sweezy, *Internal Family Systems Therapy*, 2nd ed. (New York: Guilford, 2020), 45.

4 Richard C. Schwartz, *Internal Family Systems Therapy* (New York: Guilford, 1995).

5 Susan McConnell, "Embodying the Internal Family," in *Internal Family Systems Therapy: New Dimensions,* ed. Martha Sweezy and Ellen L. Ziskind (New York: Routledge, 2013), 90–106.

Chapter 1

1 Schwartz and Sweezy, *Internal Family Systems Therapy,* 65.

2 Schwartz and Sweezy, *Internal Family Systems Therapy,* 255.

3 Linda Hartley, *Wisdom of the Body Moving* (Berkeley, CA: North Atlantic Books, 1995), xxxiii.

4 Susan Aposhyan, *Body-Mind Psychotherapy: Principles, Techniques, and Practical Applications* (New York: Norton, 2004).

Chapter 2

1 Daniel J. Siegel, *Aware: The Science and Practice of Presence* (New York: Random House, 2018).

2 Siegel, *Aware,* 75.

3 Stephen W. Porges, "Neuroception: A Subconscious System for Detecting Threats and Safety," *Zero to Three* 24, no. 5 (May 2004).

4 Deane Juhan, *Job's Body: A Handbook for Bodywork* (Barrytown, NY: Station Hill, 1987).

5 Siegel, *Aware*, 19.

6 Siegel, *Aware*, 161.

7 Bessel van der Kolk, *The Body Keeps the Score: Brain, Mind and Body in the Healing of Trauma* (New York: Viking, 2014), 100.

8 van der Kolk, *Body Keeps the Score*, 101.

9 Antonio Damasio, *The Strange Order of Things* (New York: Pantheon, 2018), 154.

10 van der Kolk, *Body Keeps the Score*, 287.

Chapter 3

1 Lynne McTaggart, *The Field: The Quest for the Secret Force of the Universe* (New York: HarperCollins, 2002).

2 Shunryu Suzuki, *Zen Mind, Beginner's Mind: Informal Talks on Zen Meditation and Practice* (New York: Weatherhill, 1970), 13.

3 Blandine Calais-Germain, *Anatomy of Breathing* (Seattle: Eastland, 2006).

4 Deb Dana, *The Polyvagal Theory in Therapy: Engaging the Rhythm of Regulation* (New York: Norton, 2018), 35.

5 Aposhyan, *Body-Mind Psychotherapy*, 128–29.

Chapter 4

1 Peter Wohlleben, *The Hidden Life of Trees: What They Feel, How They Communicate—Discoveries from a Secret World*, trans. Jane Billinghurst (Vancouver: Greystone Books, 2016).

2 Emilie Conrad, *Life on Land: The Story of Continuum* (Berkeley, CA: North Atlantic Books, 2007), 290.

3 Wilhelm Reich, *Character Analysis*, 3rd ed. (New York: Farrar, Straus and Giroux, 1949).

4 Carl Jung, *The Undiscovered Self (Present and Future)* (New York: American Library, 1959).

5 Stanley Keleman, *Your Body Speaks Its Mind* (Berkeley, CA: Center, 1981).

6 Allan Schore, *Affect Regulation and the Origin of the Self: The Neurobiology of Emotional Development* (New York: Routledge, 2003).

7 Laurie Carr, Marco Iacoboni, Marie-Charlotte Dubeau, John C. Mazziotta, and Gian Luigi Lenzi, "Neural Mechanisms of Empathy in Humans: A Relay from Neural Systems for Imitation to Limbic Areas," *PNAS* 100, no. 9 (April 29, 2003), 5497–5502, https://doi.org/10.1073/pnas.0935845100.

8 Rupert Sheldrake, *The Presence of the Past: Morphic Resonance and the Habits of Nature* (New York: Times Books, 1988).

9 Bonnie Bainbridge Cohen, *Sensing, Feeling, and Action: The Experiential Anatomy of Body-Mind Centering* (Northampton, MA: Contact Editions, 1993), 15.

10 Daniel J. Siegel, *The Mindful Therapist* (New York: Norton, 2010), 54–57.

11 Siegel, *Mindful Therapist*, 57.

12 Daniel J. Siegel, *The Developing Mind: How Relationships and the Brain Interact to Shape Who We Are*, 2nd ed. (New York: Guilford, 2012), 171.

13 Jack Kornfield, *The Wise Heart: A Guide to the Universal Teachings of Buddhist Psychology* (New York: Random House, 2008), 17.

14 Thomas Lewis, Fari Amini, and Richard Lannon, *A General Theory of Love* (New York: Random House, 2000), 63.

15 Lewis, Amini, and Lannon, *General Theory of Love*, 64.

16 Hartley, *Wisdom of the Body Moving*, 271.

17 Bainbridge Cohen, *Sensing, Feeling, and Action*, 15.

18 Bruce H. Lipton, *The Biology of Belief: Unleashing the Power of Consciousness, Matter and Miracles* (New York: Hay House, 2005).

19 Candace Pert, *Molecules of Emotion: The Science Behind Mind-Body Medicine* (New York: Touchstone, 1997).

20 Paul Pearsall, *The Heart's Code: Tapping the Wisdom and Power of Our Heart Energy* (New York: Broadway Books, 1998).

21 James Doty, *Into the Magic Shop: A Neurosurgeon's Quest to Discover the Mysteries of the Brain and the Secrets of the Heart* (New York: Penguin, 2017).

22 Joseph LeDoux, *Synaptic Self: How Our Brains Become Who We Are* (London: Macmillan, 2003), 324.

23 Allan Schore, *Right Brain Psychotherapy* (New York: Norton, 2019).

Chapter 5

1 Charles Darwin, *The Expression of the Emotions in Man and Animals* (London: Oxford University Press, 1998). First published 1872.

2 van der Kolk, *Body Keeps the Score*, 236.

3 van der Kolk, *Body Keeps the Score*, 209.

4 Juhan, *Job's Body*, 114.

5 Mabel Elsworth Todd, *The Thinking Body: A Study of the Balancing Forces of Dynamic Man* (New York: Paul B. Hoeber, 1937), 31.

6 Dana, *Polyvagal Theory in Therapy*.

7 Susan Cahill, "Tapestry of a Clinician: Blending Authentic Movement and the Internal Family Systems Model," *Journal of Dance and Somatic Practices* 7, no. 2 (2015), 251.

8 Peter Levine, *Waking the Tiger: Healing Trauma* (Berkeley, CA: North Atlantic Books, 1997).

9 Bainbridge Cohen, *Sensing, Feeling, and Action.*

10 Hartley, *Wisdom of the Body Moving,* 27.

11 Aposhyan, *Body-Mind Psychotherapy,* 205.

12 Ann L. Sinko, "Legacy Burdens," in *Innovations and Elaborations in Internal Family Systems Therapy,* ed. M. Sweezy and Ellen L. Ziskind (Oxford, UK: Routledge, 2016).

Chapter 6

1 Mic Hunter and Jim Struve, *The Ethical Use of Touch in Psychotherapy* (London: Sage, 1997).

2 Sharon Heller, *The Vital Touch: How Intimate Contact with Your Baby Leads to Happier, Healthier Development* (New York: Henry Holt, 1997).

3 Ofer Zur and Nola Nordmarken, "To Touch or Not to Touch: Exploring the Myth of Prohibition on Touch in Psychotherapy and Counseling," Zur Institute, accessed February 19, 2020, www.zurinstitute.com/touch-in-therapy/.

4 Sidney Jourard, "An Exploratory Study of Body-Accessibility," *British Journal of Social and Clinical Psychology* 5, no. 3 (1966), 221–31.

5 Ashley Montagu, *Touching: The Human Significance of the Skin* (New York: Harper & Row, 1971).

6 Bainbridge Cohen, *Sensing, Feeling, and Action.*

7 Adam Gopnik, "Feel Me: What the New Science of Touch Says About Ourselves," *New Yorker,* May 9, 2016.

8 Aline LaPierre, "From Felt-Sense to Felt-Self: Neuroaffective Touch and the Relational Matrix," *Psychologist-Psychoanalyst* 23, no. 4 (2003).

9 Juhan, *Job's Body.*

10 Juhan, *Job's Body,* 182.

11 Tiffany Field, *Touch* (Cambridge, MA: MIT Press, 2001).

12 Zur and Nordmarken, "To Touch or Not to Touch: Exploring the Myth of Prohibition on Touch in Psychotherapy and Counseling."

13 Montagu, *Touching,* 46.

14 James W. Prescott, "Body Pleasure and the Origins of Violence," *Bulletin of the Atomic Scientists,* November 1975, pp. 10–20, www.violence.de/prescott/bulletin/article.html.

15 Edward W. L. Smith, Pauline Rose Clance, and Suzanne Imes, eds., *Touch in Psychotherapy: Theory, Research and Practice* (New York: Guilford, 1998).

16 Babette Rothschild, *The Body Remembers: The Psychophysiology of Trauma and Trauma Treatment* (New York: Norton, 2000).

17 van der Kolk, *Body Keeps the Score,* 215–17.

18 Courtenay Young, "Doing Effective Body-Psychotherapy Without Touch," *Energy & Character,* no. 34 (September 2005), 50–60, www.courtenay-young.co.uk /courtenay/articles/B-P_without_Touch_1.pdf.

19 Lynn Ungar, "Pandemic," March 11, 2020, www.lynnungar.com/poems/pandemic.

Chapter 7

1 Mariel Pastor with Dick Schwartz, "The Unburdened Internal System," 2012, www.marielpastor.com/the-unburdened-system.

2 Schwartz and Sweezy, *Internal Family Systems Therapy,* 251.

3 Schwartz and Sweezy, *Internal Family Systems Therapy,* 252.

4 Malcolm W. Browne, "Far Apart, 2 Particles Respond Faster Than Light," *New York Times,* July 22, 1997, http://nytimes.com/1997/07/22/science/far-apart-2 -particles-respond-faster-than-light.html.

5 Heinz Pagels, *The Cosmic Code: Quantum Physics as the Language of Nature* (New York: Simon & Schuster, 1982), 349.

6 Shahram Shiva, trans., *Rumi, Thief of Sleep: 180 Quatrains from the Persian* (Prescott, AZ: Hohm Press, 2000). All Rumi quotations are from this volume.

7 Jack Kornfield, *After the Ecstasy, the Laundry: How the Heart Grows Wise on the Spiritual Path* (New York: Bantam, 2000.

8 Jack Kornfield, *The Art of Forgiveness, Lovingkindness, and Peace* (New York: Random House, 2002), 185.

9 Rainer Maria Rilke, *Rilke's Book of Hours: Love Poems to God,* trans. Anita Barrows and Joanna Macy (New York: Berkley Publishing, 1996).

10 Schwartz and Sweezy, *Internal Family Systems Therapy,* 42.

11 Jorge N. Ferrer, *Revisioning Transpersonal Theory: A Participatory Vision of Human Spirituality* (Albany: State University of New York Press, 2002).

Index

About the Author

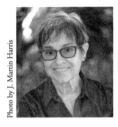

Photo by J. Martin Harris

SUSAN MCCONNELL, MA, CHT, has been teaching Internal Family Systems in the US and internationally since 1997. As the founding developer of Somatic IFS, Susan offers retreats and trainings in embodying the internal system with applications for all clinical issues.

About North Atlantic Books

NORTH ATLANTIC BOOKS (NAB) is an independent, nonprofit publisher committed to a bold exploration of the relationships between mind, body, spirit, and nature. Founded in 1974, NAB aims to nurture a holistic view of the arts, sciences, humanities, and healing. To make a donation or to learn more about our books, authors, events, and newsletter, please visit www.northatlanticbooks.com.